T0137636

BEAUTY BY DESIGN

BEAUTY BY DESIGN

The Artistry of Plastic Surgery

Illustrations By: Anne Marie Johnson
and Ronie Pios

**Malcolm W. Marks;
Christopher A. Park**

Copyright © 2016 by Malcolm W. Marks; Christopher A. Park.

Library of Congress Control Number:		2016902704
ISBN:	Hardcover	978-1-5144-6771-8
	Softcover	978-1-5144-6772-5
	eBook	978-1-5144-6773-2

All rights reserved. No part of this book may be reproduced or transmitted in any form or by any means, electronic or mechanical, including photocopying, recording, or by any information storage and retrieval system, without permission in writing from the copyright owner.

Any people depicted in stock imagery provided by Thinkstock are models, and such images are being used for illustrative purposes only.
Certain stock imagery © Thinkstock.

The information provided in this book is designed to provide helpful information on the subjects discussed. This book is not meant to be used, nor should it be used, to diagnose or treat any medical or plastic surgery condition. For diagnosis or treatment of any plastic surgery problem, consult your own plastic surgeon. The publisher and author are not responsible for any specific health or surgical needs that may require medical supervision and are not liable for any damages or negative consequences from any treatment, action, application or preparation, to any person reading or following the information in this book. References are provided for informational purposes only and do not constitute endorsement of any websites or other sources. Readers should be aware that the websites listed in this book may change.

Print information available on the last page.

Rev. date: 08/04/2016

To order additional copies of this book, contact:
Xlibris
1-888-795-4274
www.Xlibris.com
Orders@Xlibris.com
703077

To the patients, staff, and students interested in learning about and refining their knowledge of cosmetic surgery.

—Malcolm

To my patients and those others seeking to understand more about plastic surgery: where the combination of science, medicine, anatomy, art, and beauty meet, and the application to each individual repair of the physical form keeps me challenged, stimulated, and excited.

—Chris

ACKNOWLEDGMENTS

Both Dr. Park and Dr. Marks wish to acknowledge those who made this publication a reality, including Anne Marie Johnson, illustrator at Vivo Visuals, and Sandra Binford, our editor.

Dr. Marks wishes to acknowledge all those who have inspired him in his career, foremost, his father Charles Marks, extraordinary physician, educator and author. He also wishes to acknowledge all those who have shared their knowledge and skills during his training and career, and to the residents and students who have stimulated him to try to be as talented as they will be. He is especially grateful to his wife Sharon and children: Kevin, Lara, Eric, & Nicole for their enduring love and support.

Dr. Park wishes to acknowledge those who have participated in his plastic-surgery education, which include the coauthor, Dr. Malcolm Marks; as well as Dr. Lou Argenta; Dr. Anthony Defranzo; Dr. Lisa David; Dr. Joe Molnar; and Dr. Jim Thompson at Wake Forest University; Dr. Luis Vasconez, who is the mentor who inspired him to choose plastic surgery as a career; his clinical staff; and his family, who supports him and understands how work and this endeavor may take some of his time away from them, but not his love, particularly his wife, Elizabeth, and his children, Ashley and Alden.

CONTENTS

INTRODUCTION

We are fortunate to live in a golden age of health care. A wonderful array of technological and medical advances can keep us alive for many more years than in the past. For many, though, it is not enough just to add years of life. We need to be both productive during those added years and capable of competing with younger people in the workplace. We have to develop a sense of well-being and satisfy our own individual ideals of physical appearance. Ideally, we are not excessively vain and are satisfied with our appearance. It is, however, understandable to develop an interest in maintaining and improving our physical appearance while developing an internal equanimity. It is to these seekers that we dedicate this book.

The mystery of the aging process is unraveling. As life expectancy has increased dramatically in the past half century, we have learned that longevity and good health are associated. Moreover, we know that long life can be matched with continued enjoyment of existence: these two are not mutually exclusive, so we can have both. Such hope is enhanced by the knowledge that most people live well beyond one hundred years of age in certain parts of the world, notably in Abkhazia in Georgia (formerly part of the Soviet Union), Hunza in the Kashmir, and Vilcabamba in Ecuador.

Long before advanced age is reached, the early signs of senescence begin to appear: Wrinkles form around the eyes and mouth, the nose becomes longer and wider, the cheeks and jowls sag, bags appear under the eyes, and the skin loses its elasticity. Hair becomes thinner and grayer, the earlobes lengthen, and age spots appear. Vision is no longer sharp, and farsightedness increases. Women lose up to 1½" in height, while men may lose up to 2½" in height.

Research has discovered many causes for aging and proposed different reasons for them. Many of these ideas are covered in the news media and in health magazines: Damage by oxygen free radicals, cells of the body not being able to divide forever, programmed destruction of cells by "aging hormones," and so forth. There are also changes in the heart and lungs, metabolism, immunity, and hormones.

Despite this chronicle of physical deterioration, individuals need not feel a sense of helplessness—victims of the aging process. Although we accept that aging is inevitable, we need to emphasize that we may have the capability to control the rate of our bodies' aging by taking care of them. Long life should not mean keeping just ahead of chronic illness by controlling medical problems like high blood sugar, high blood pressure, and failure of major organs. In order to preserve physical function, we should not smoke, we should eat regular and nutritious meals, and we should stay within 20% of the weight recommended for our age, gender, and height. We should engage in moderate aerobic exercise (ideally three times a week) and limit our consumption of alcohol. We should, whenever possible, get enough sleep and minimize stress in our daily lives.

People resist the relentless progression of physical decline that seems to be the price of longevity. While mental and physical activities are enhanced by good nutrition and healthful behavior, advances in medical care can help lead to a happy, healthy, and long life. The modern medical interventions now available to keep us looking young are no less than amazing.

Cosmetic Surgery Statistics

There has been a significant increase in the number of cosmetic surgery procedures in the United States over the past two decades. Statistics released by the American Society of Plastic Surgeons report almost 1.7 million cosmetic surgery operations performed by its members in 2014. This is a 300% increase since 1996.

The most common surgical procedure is breast augmentation; the next most common procedures are rhinoplasty (nose reshaping), liposuction, eyelid surgery, face-lift and abdominoplasty (tummy tuck). The most common initial complaint, however, is facial aging. Fewer face-lifts are being performed now than a decade ago because minimally invasive procedures (6.7 million in 2014 in patients age 40–54) are available to manage facial wrinkling: fillers, botulinum toxin, cellulite treatment, chemical peels, and laser services (see table).

Men now account for 13% of all individuals seeking cosmetic surgery and 8% of those seeking minimally invasive surgery. There has also been an increase in younger people seeking cosmetic surgery operations. Among all age categories, nearly half (49%) of patients are between forty and fifty-four years old (see table I-I).

Table I-I. Cosmetic, Minimally Invasive Procedures among Patients Aged 40–54 in 2014[a]

Procedure	2014 Total[b]	Percentage of procedures by 40–54 yo
Botox	**3,813,032**	57
Cellulite treatment	7,007	24
Chemical peel	**526,499**	42
Laser hair removal	**403,548**	36
Laser skin resurfacing	220,526	41
Laser treatment of leg veins	63,118	30
Microdermabrasion	**387,131**	44
Sclerotherapy	158,844	49
Soft-tissue fillers	1,126,662	49
Calcium hydroxyapatite (Radiesse)	101,360	39
Collagen	7,899	36
Fat	22,971	34
Hyaluronic acid (Juvéderm line, Restylane line, Perlane)	**918,296**	51
Polylactic acid (Sculptra)	76,136	57
Total Cosmetic, Minimally Invasive Procedures	**6,706,367**	**50**

[a]   Figures represent procedures performed in the United States by plastic surgeons and other physicians who are certified by boards that are recognized by the American Board of Medical Specialties.

[b]   Top five procedures in bold and red.

[c]   Figures do not add up to 100% because patients may choose more than one procedure.

[d]   Botox data reflect number of anatomic sites injected.

Table modified from the American Society of Plastic Surgeons. *2015 Report of the 2014 Statistics: National Clearinghouse of Plastic Surgery Statistics* [Internet]. Arlington Heights, IL: American Society of Plastic Surgeons; 2015.

Table I-II. Number and Percentages of Cosmetic Surgery Procedures by Gender in 2014[a]

	Gender	
Procedure Category	**Women**	**Men**
Surgical	1,364,103	204,611
Minimally invasive	13,306,320	1,057,192
Total	14,875,034 (92%)	1,261,803 (8%)

[a] All figures are projected and approximate. Figures represent procedures performed in the United States by plastic surgeons and other physicians who are certified by boards that are recognized by the American Board of Medical Specialties.

Source data from the American Society of Plastic Surgeons. *2015 Report of the 2014 Statistics: National Clearinghouse of Plastic Surgery Statistics* [Internet]. Arlington Heights, IL: American Society of Plastic Surgeons; 2015.

Achieving Happiness with the Human Form

As commendable as the desire for self-improvement may be, there is a danger that the concept of beauty can become an obsession rather than a realistic goal. Vanity may lead someone to an unhealthy extreme. It is possible to make specific features of the face more attractive yet make the entire face less attractive than ever. This may result in a situation where the ultimate lack of symmetry is unattractive rather than beautiful or pleasing. No surgery can cure emptiness of the soul; instead, it may convert an unhappy individual with a blemished appearance to a physically attractive person who remains unhappy.

It is essential that during the consultation between physician and patient, excessive expectation be curbed and pragmatic reality defined. If the physician fails to understand the problems inherent in a patient's psyche, the patient will be dissatisfied with the end result. No matter how satisfactory the anatomical outcome, if the patient harbors an unspoken desire for total transformation to an undefined and life-changing ideal, the surgery will be a failure.

It is obvious from the numbers of people desiring cosmetic surgery that some individuals base the pursuit of happiness on physical attractiveness. Through surgery, individuals seek to attain the opposites of their existing realities: The bald person desires scalp hair, the small-breasted woman aspires to have larger breasts, and the large-breasted woman prefers smaller dimensions. The person with too large, too small, or otherwise perceived abnormalities of the nose seeks happiness through the appropriate surgical corrections of the nose (nose reshaping). Those with excessive fat seek either liposuction or procedures to remove excess tissue, like those done in a tummy tuck. Even transsexual procedures are available to induce happiness in the man or woman who is unhappy with the existing gender.

Training and Qualifications in Plastic Surgery

The patient and the public may feel that happiness may be brought about by "simple" cosmetic surgery, but the doctor has a different point of view. The cosmetic surgeon's techniques are not different from ones used in other reconstructive operations such as breast restoration after mastectomy for breast cancer or nose reconstruction after trauma. It is therefore important to know that your doctor, who may provide "cosmetic" services, is fully trained in the many skills of plastic and reconstructive surgery.

Locating the appropriate cosmetic surgeon can be a daunting task. Ideally, the doctor to whom one plans to trust his or her well-being will be wise, well educated, competent, and confident. Whether the doctor is well trained, safe, and competent can be hard to know, and many referrals are purely word of mouth. But even in that scenario, a specific patient may not know a particular surgeon's ability to perform the specific surgical procedure or procedures that they want.

Confusing the public even more, any doctor can call himself a cosmetic surgeon regardless of his training. He may be a good and well-trained cosmetic surgeon, but there is no requirement to have training or experience when claiming to be a cosmetic surgeon. Less often is the term *plastic surgeon* abused, but it can be as well. Trade laws in the United States allow licensed medical doctors to practice any kind of medicine they choose. As doctors receive lower reimbursement from insurance companies and other third parties for medically necessary treatments, many physicians are trying to augment their income by adding cosmetic treatments, including spa services, injectables, and even cosmetic surgery, all of which are usually paid by the patient in full before the operation begins. There are many physicians doing so with little more than a weekend course or limited peer-to-peer training rather than true medical specialty training. Another reason that this scenario is increasing is that most of the review and controls on physicians are peer-driven through hospitals or colleagues. Cosmetic surgery, however, can be an office-based practice where there may be no oversight. As scary as this sounds, it is true that there is no required review of the doctor's qualifications and no peers ably challenge a surgeon to keep to acceptable surgical and safety standards. As a result, unqualified physicians can continue to operate within their own offices as long as the patients come in. Although the physicians could lose their medical license if enough concerns were raised by patients, the physician avoids any peer review of their abilities in decision making, technical ability, and appropriate patient care. The vast majority of plastic surgeons and even other physicians who practice cosmetic surgery within their offices are qualified to do so, but the individual patients must research to understand whether they should trust their future cosmetic success to the surgeons they may consider. A person who is working to choose a qualified doctor for any specific kind of surgery should check on four areas: (1) training and board certification, (2) membership in well-recognized societies of peer surgeons, (3) hospital privileges, and (4) experience. The available safeguards below should give readers the insight, tools, and knowledge necessary to research and select a cosmetic surgeon.

Board Certification

While finding a doctor with board certification is no guarantee of having a successful surgical outcome, it is an important criterion in evaluating a doctor's background. The existence of various boards and societies proves that many different types of physicians have an interest and expertise in cosmetic procedures. It is important to realize, however, that the doctors may have received training that is very narrow in scope. That means that some doctors may not have the exact training required by the surgery the patient wants.

Some boards are sanctioned only by their own members, so patients should look for a meaningful certification from a board that is recognized by the American Board of Medical Specialties. To earn this level of certification, doctors must complete a multiple-year training period or residency in a specialty after leaving medical school. They must then pass both written and oral examinations.

Authoritative medical boards that have major interests in cosmetic surgery are the American Board of Plastic Surgery, the American Board of Otolaryngology, the American Board of Ophthalmology, and the American Board of Dermatology.

The American Board of Plastic Surgery

Doctors who are certified by the American Board of Plastic Surgery have completed at least six years of full-time surgical training and practice after medical school. They have, at a minimum, three years of general-surgery training, two years of plastic-surgery training in an accredited training program in an accredited hospital facility, and one additional year of practice after training. They also must have passed examinations in plastic and reconstructive surgery.

The training program is devoted to reconstructive and cosmetic surgical procedures involving the entire body in patients of all ages. Training includes surgeries of the face, head, neck, breasts, skin, trunk, and extremities. Some plastic and reconstructive surgeons choose to complete a fellowship in cosmetic surgery, but such programs do not provide an official Certificate of Additional Qualification for this subspecialty.

Other Specialty Medical Boards

The American Board of Otolaryngology

The American Board of Otolaryngology certifies doctors of the ears, nose, and throat. It requires at least five years of surgical training at an accredited program in an accredited hospital. The cosmetic training is devoted to surgery of the face, head, and neck areas. Otolaryngologists may also pursue an additional fellowship in facial plastic surgery.

The American Board of Ophthalmology

This board certifies doctors who treat diseases and deformities of the eye. Training requires a minimum of five years at an accredited program in an accredited hospital facility. The training is devoted to diseases and surgery of the eye and structures around the eye.

The American Board of Dermatology

Doctors who are sanctioned by the American Board of Dermatology have undergone a three-year residency training in an accredited hospital. The training focuses entirely on treatment of diseases of the skin. There is not major surgical training, but most programs will train the dermatologist to remove skin cancers or lesions and to complete other office-based procedures.

Otolaryngologists, ophthalmologists, and dermatologists who are interested in general cosmetic surgery usually seek further training in plastic surgery after completing the proper training to earn their initial board certifications. Membership in these certain professional societies reflects these doctors' professional standing and reputation, so patients should research a surgeon's training history and current society memberships.

Cosmetic Surgery Societies

Large societies that cosmetic surgeons may join are nationwide and often use the titles American Association or American Society. There are also state and local medical societies and societies for specific specialties. These societies can give doctors a wealth of information, but the management and reliability of these regional entities can certainly vary. A patient cannot be sure that a surgeon has specific ability or experience because he or she holds membership in a local society.

The American Society of Plastic Surgery

This is the leading society of plastic and reconstructive surgeons. In order to be eligible to join, a doctor must have both board certification in plastic and reconstructive surgery and a formal review of clinical experience by peer surgeons. In addition, member surgeons must regularly complete continuing medical education and adhere to a strict code of ethics.

Other Specialty Medical Societies

The American Association of Facial Plastic and Reconstructive Surgeons

Members of this association must have board certification that is recognized by the American Board of Otolaryngology. They also must have a proven clinical experience in facial plastic and reconstructive surgery. Members of the American Association of Facial Plastic and Reconstructive Surgeons should have interest and experience in cosmetic surgeries of the face. However, they probably will not have received training in breast surgery, contouring procedures, liposuction of the body, or other cosmetic procedures beyond the face.

American Society of Dermatologic Surgeons

Dermatologic surgeons have completed dermatology training and are board-certified by the American Board of Dermatology. While a regular dermatologist is not trained in surgery, a dermatologic surgeon has received additional training in surgical techniques to treat the skin and associated skin problems. A dermatologic surgeon is trained to remove skin cancers and tumors. Some of them also have limited training in cosmetic surgery procedures.

American Society of Ophthalmic Plastic and Reconstructive Surgery

Ophthalmologists can choose to train in oculoplastic surgery, a specialty devoted to cosmetic and reconstructive procedures of the eyes and surrounding structures of the orbit. Many oculoplastic surgeons learn other cosmetic surgery techniques in a hands-on situation and have little formal training in some of these procedures before beginning their practices. A patient must be careful to discern the amount of experience an oculoplastic surgeon has in treating a specific problem that is not located in the eye or orbit.

Experience

Clearly, the level of a doctor's experience may be difficult to determine at the consultation. Even if good education was completed during training, it can be nearly impossible for the patient to know how important that education is. A veteran plastic surgeon will have refined his techniques, whereas a young, well-trained plastic surgeon may know new modifications and techniques for each procedure.

It is reasonable for the patient to ask the surgeon these questions: (1) "How long have you been performing this particular operation?" (2) "How many have you done?" and (3) "When did you last do this procedure?" An ethical surgeon will be honest about his or her experience and comfort with a given procedure.

Using Specialty Directories

Because of its leading position among cosmetic surgery societies, the authors place the utmost confidence in the information services provided by the American Society of Plastic Surgeons. The society will provide the names of five plastic surgeons in a general geographic area who are qualified to perform a particular operation. Because those surgeons belong to the American Society of Plastic and Reconstructive Surgery, it is certain that they are also board-certified in plastic and reconstructive surgery, have had a minimum of three years of surgical training, and have completed a further two or more years of cosmetic and reconstructive surgical training involving the face and the rest of the body. The society can be contacted at its toll-free physician-referral number, 1-888-4-PLASTIC (1-888-475-2784) or online at www.plasticsurgery.org.

A surgeon's credentials can also be checked in the *Compendium of Certified Medical Specialists*, a publication of the American Board of Medical Specialties, by phone at 1-866-275-2267 or online at www.abms. org. This is the final and probably the most important credential check a patient can make.

When checking credentials as outlined above, it is important that the patient understands specifically what training a physician's board certification covers and for what procedures has the surgeon been trained. An ocular plastic surgeon should limit surgical practice to the eye, eyelids, and orbit. An otolaryngologist should limit practice to the head and neck.

A dermatologist, or dermatologic surgeon, should offer procedures only at the level of the skin, while a surgeon certified by the American Board of Plastic Surgery may offer all forms of cosmetic surgery. The physician should have specific experience in the procedure the patient actually wants. The physician should have privileges at an accredited hospital to perform that procedure, whether they plan to use a hospital facility or not. Ideally, the surgeon chosen will have been recommended by a physician or friends who have had experience with that doctor and will be a member of the American Society of Plastic Surgeons.

Hospital Privileges

If training and abilities are proven, a hospital after careful review may grant a doctor surgical privileges for specific procedures. While not all plastic surgeons continue to use hospitals and therefore hospital privileges should not be viewed as a requirement, one way to know whether a surgeon has training in a particular procedure is to confirm that the surgeon has privileges to do the same procedure in a hospital. If a patient is researching an office-based surgeon, it is important to verify that a hospital did not cancel the surgeon's privileges for cause or practice-based reason.

Accredited Hospital or Surgery Center (ASC)

Even if a surgeon has privileges, the hospital or surgical facility itself must also be accredited. Accreditation certifies that the surgical facility maintains a standard of safety and undergoes regular inspections. The American Society of Plastic Surgery requires its members to perform surgeries in an accredited facility. If a surgery is to be performed in a physician's office, the patient must make certain that the surgical suite is in an accredited surgical center. Accreditation certifies that the surgical facility maintains a standard of safety and undergoes regular inspections.

A facility may be accredited by any one of the following groups:

- The American Association for Accreditation for Ambulatory Surgery Facilities (AAAASF at www.aaaasf.org)
- Accreditation Association for Ambulatory Health Care (AAAHC at www.aaahc.org)

- The Joint Commission (www.JointCommission.org), formerly known as the Joint Commission on Accreditation of Health Care Organizations (JCAHO)
- Medicare

Certification will ensure that the surgical facility has the appropriate staffing, medical equipment, peer review among surgical providers, and record-keeping.

Choosing a Plastic Surgeon

Referral

The most common way people choose a plastic surgeon is through a recommendation from a trusted physician or friend. A patient should have reasonable confidence in a referral from a physician who has seen other patients before and after surgical procedures and can therefore provide an educated opinion. A patient can ask whether the physician would trust the surgeon to operate on him- or herself, a family member, or one of his patients.

Personal referrals are subject to much more bias than a physician referral is. Someone else's experiences do not necessarily reflect the usual experience that patients have with a particular plastic surgeon. However, cumulative comments, good or bad, can suggest a trend.

The Consult

A patient must feel comfortable and be able to communicate with the surgeon. A frank, open discussion ensures that the surgeon clearly understands the patient's desires and motivations for seeking surgery and assures the surgeon that the patient has reasonable expectations. In return, the surgeon needs the knowledge and interpersonal skills to clearly explain recommendations and how the surgical techniques can achieve the desired goals.

The doctor should act professionally. The office environment should create an aura of competence that makes patients feel comfortable and secure. The doctor should be willing and easily able to answer questions and should patiently explain things that patients may not fully understand, for example, the details of a procedure and its potential risks and complications. The doctor may show pre- and postoperative (before and after) photographs to help demonstrate results, but these are examples of individual patients' experiences, not guarantees of a good outcome—the doctor is not likely to show disappointing results or complications. Many doctors are reluctant to use other patients' photographs to sell the operation, so they will prefer not to show photographs. This is not because they have limited experience. In any case, red flags should be raised in the mind of any patient who consults a doctor who becomes upset or frustrated with these questions or who evades discussing them openly and frankly.

Patients should be wary of the surgeon who finds a multitude of other procedures to do or things to fix. While a doctor should not lead patients toward procedures in which they have no interest, patients should be open to suggestions. For example, a patient may desire liposuction of the abdomen and find the doctor leading the discussion toward the more invasive abdominoplasty. The surgeon may be suggesting a more aggressive operation because his or her clinical experience shows that it is needed to achieve the desired result. In other situations, however, the doctor should be just as willing to recommend a smaller procedure when an excessive procedure is requested. Consider the example above: a patient may arrive and immediately request a tummy tuck when only liposuction is needed.

Anesthesia

Most cosmetic procedures require anesthesia. Some minor procedures can be done with topical (skin-level) or local anesthesia. Topical anesthesia has two disadvantages: it requires a delay after application, and it is usually unable to block sensation or feeling completely. Local anesthesia is given by injection either along the path of a major nerve (this is called a nerve block) or locally around the surgical site. There are a variety of chemicals with different timelines of onset and duration. The anesthetic mixture may include diluted epinephrine (adrenaline); this increases the amount of time the nerve block works and decreases blood flow, which reduces the loss of blood during surgery. Unfortunately, long-acting local anesthetics take longer to begin working.

If true sedation is required, an anesthesia provider may be called to assist. This may be an anesthesiologist (who is a physician) or a nurse anesthetist (CRNA), depending on the preference of the surgeon, state or hospital rules, and regional trends. Using an anesthesiologist carries obvious benefits but usually at significantly higher cost. Nurse anesthetists are usually well trained and comfortable with all sedation techniques.

The different levels of sedation that are frequently used are oral sedation, intravenous sedation, monitored anesthesia care (deep sedation with natural breathing), and general anesthesia that requires artificial ventilation. These are escalating levels of sedation that require increasing numbers of monitoring and safety provisions. It is usually possible to provide the first three options in a variety of settings, including the physician's office, but the ability to use general anesthesia depends upon state rules and usually requires the surgery to take place at an accredited surgical facility.

Cost of Cosmetic Surgery

The costs of cosmetic surgery procedures are rarely covered by insurance companies. They are entirely borne by the patient. Cosmetic surgery procedures usually must be paid in full ahead of time. The costs of an operation include the surgeon's fee, the operating-room costs, and if required, the cost of a nurse or physician anesthetist, the cost of any implants, and the cost of an overnight hospital stay. Table I-III shows typical surgeons' fees for the most common cosmetic operations. It does not display other fees, such as facility fees, anesthesia fees, recovery fees, or implant fees.

Table I-III. Average Surgeon/Physician Fees for Surgical and Minimally Invasive Cosmetic Procedures in the United States in 2014[a]

Surgical Procedure	Fee
Breast augmentation (augmentation mammaplasty)	$3,708
Breast implant removals (augmentation patients only)	$2,330
Breast lift (mastopexy)	$4,377
Breast reduction in men (gynecomastia)	$3,333
Buttock implants Buttock fat grafting	$4,580 $4,077
Buttock lift	$4,509
Calf augmentation	$3,315
Cheek implant (malar augmentation)	$2,651
Chin augmentation (mentoplasty)	$2,085
Dermabrasion	$1,150
Ear surgery (otoplasty)	$2,963
Eyelid surgery (blepharoplasty)	$2,874
Face-lift (rhytidectomy)	$6,550
Forehead lift	$3,201
Hair transplantation	$5,845
Lip augmentation (other than injectable materials)	$1,606
Liposuction	$2,971
Lower-body lift	$7,843
Nose reshaping (rhinoplasty)	$4,694
Pectoral implants	$4,312
Thigh lift	$4,653
Tummy tuck (abdominoplasty)	$5,493

Upper-arm lift	$3,936
Minimally Invasive Procedure	**Fee**
Botulinum toxin	$371
Cellulite treatment	$291
Chemical peel	$632
Laser hair removal	$289
Laser skin resurfacing	
Ablative	$2,146
Nonablative (fractionated laser, etc.)	$1,062
Laser treatment of leg veins	$344
Microdermabrasion	$143
Sclerotherapy	$347
Soft-tissue fillers	
Calcium hydroxyapatite (Radiesse)	$623
Fat	$1,791
Polylactic acid (Sculptra)	$778
Hyaluronic acid (Restylane line, Juvéderm line, Perlane)	$590
Polymethyl-methacrylate microspheres (e.g., Artefill)	$867

[a]   Average of surgeons fees only. Fees generally vary according to region of country and patient needs. Fees do not include anesthesia, operating-room facilities, or other related expenses. Figures represent fees for procedures performed in the United States by plastic surgeons and other physicians who are certified by boards that are recognized by the American Board of Medical Specialties.

Table modified from the American Society of Plastic Surgeons. *2015 Report of the 2014 Statistics: National Clearinghouse of Plastic Surgery Statistics* [Internet]. Arlington Heights, IL: American Society of Plastic Surgeons; 2015.

Costs for different procedures vary widely according to the geographic location, practice location, and physician background. The same operation is probably considerably more expensive in Manhattan or Beverly Hills than in a small town in the Midwest or Southeast. The most important factor in selecting a doctor remains the quality and reputation of the physician, but patients certainly can shop around and compare rates.

In some areas, a teaching hospital with a plastic surgery resident's clinic may offer cosmetic surgery at a significant discount. Patients may save over 50% of usual fees in such a hospital. The consultations, operation, and postoperative care are done by a senior resident in plastic surgery. These trainees are generally highly trained surgeons who are within twelve months of going out on their own in a plastic surgery practice. They are also very well supervised by board-certified and experienced plastic surgeons who also have faculty positions at university-based medical schools. If a patient considers this option, he or she must understand all the details about who will perform the surgery and care and who is supervising the resident. Specifically, the patient must find out how much input the supervising, faculty-level surgeon will have during the operation.

Different doctors have different policies for refunds if a patient cancels a scheduled surgery. Many doctors have a policy that lists nonrefundable and partially refundable fees if you cancel surgery after a certain preoperative date unless you have a valid excuse. Some doctors work with finance companies, and their offices will assist in the application process for a loan to cover an operation.

SURGICAL CONCERNS
AND COMPLICATIONS

Preoperative
Postoperative

Preoperative Considerations

Certainly, the complex relationship between surgery and existing medical conditions is beyond the scope of this book and most patients' knowledge and must be left to the surgeon, but medical conditions can have a dramatic impact on the safety and results of cosmetic surgery and must be discussed with your surgeon.

Medications also affect surgery. There are medications that affect healing, such as steroids, autoimmune medications, and chemotherapeutic agents. There are also many medications that thin the blood and increase the risk of bleeding with surgery. Many potent oral medications are prescribed to intentionally reduce blood clotting, such as warfarin (Coumadin), aspirin, clopidogrel bisulfate (Plavix), cilostazol (Pletal), Pradaxa (dabigatran), Xarelto (rivaroxaban), and Eliquis (apixaban). But many other medications thin the blood as a side effect, including over-the-counter medications such as nonsteroidal anti-inflammatory drugs (NSAIDS, i.e., ibuprofen), aspirin, fish oil, and vitamin E. Patients who take medications that thin the blood should discuss with their physicians the risk of bleeding. It is recommended to bring a list of all medications—prescribed, herbal, and over the counter—since there are many other medications that can affect bleeding.

Nicotine in all forms has a negative impact on healing. This is in addition to the negative long-term consequences of smoking, which are well known to include cancer, atherosclerosis, and loss of skin elasticity, among others. Acutely, nicotine causes vasoconstriction of the small blood vessels in the body. Much of plastic surgery is dependent on moving, lifting, and tucking of tissues. After these procedures, it is vital for blood flow in small blood vessels, especially those right under the skin, to be intact to allow for healing without the death or infection of the tissues moved. A single dose of nicotine can cause spasm of the blood vessels for a month, so it is very important to be honest and open with the use of nicotine and to understand that there are many procedures not recommended on nicotine users.

Prior surgery or radiation also can affect surgical options. Both treatments will have altered existing tissues and blood flow. This may increase the risk, alter, or prohibit altogether, the procedure of interest. So again, open and honest communication with the surgeon is very important.

Postoperative Expectations

The most important components of a successful outcome are good communication, surgical skill, and realistic expectations. With the right outlook, cosmetic surgery can be one of the greatest events in one's life and can lead to changes in all aspects of life. However, the scalpel is not a magic wand, and the physical changes that result from surgery can serve only as a catalyst to the desired health, mental, and emotional changes that can follow.

Results should not be judged by the immediate postoperative appearance. Almost all surgical procedures are going to result in swelling and bruising, which may distort appearances. The amount of swelling, bulging, or tension is dependent on the procedure performed but may persist for weeks to months. In addition, many procedures require surgical modifications to allow for the effects of gravity, which may delay appearance of the true result for months.

The postoperative period is a challenge for the patient, and one of the most difficult concerns lies in knowing when to call the surgeon's office. We will use this section to try to alleviate some anxiety about expected postoperative changes and to elucidate worrisome problems. However, this list is not all-inclusive and should not be treated as such. If you are unsure about your recovery, it is safer to call the physician's office.

Expected Changes

Swelling

Surgery is controlled trauma to tissues with a purpose, but it is trauma nonetheless, and the body's response is inflammatory. Inflammation causes the blood vessels to become leaky so that they can deliver cells and fluid to help in the healing process. This swelling—caused by biochemical agents called mediators—is referred to as postoperative edema and may take days, weeks, and even months to resolve, depending on the extent of the procedure.

Minor drainage

Just as fluid accumulates at the surgical site from the above mechanisms, fluid may leak out of the incision site. This may be clear or blood-tinged. A small amount of blood can turn a dressing or article of clothing alarmingly red, and it can be difficult to determine the extent of bleeding on the basis of color alone. Other important factors include the shade of red, the amount of drainage, the change in amount and color, and the presence of a collection of blood in a pocket under the wound. If the color is diluted or pink, it is usually minor bleeding. Dark-red blood may signal a bleeding problem in the veins, but most commonly, it signals the approach of the clotting (hemostasis) that is needed for healing.

Altered sensation and innervation

Surgery can interrupt the roles of both sensory (touch, pain, etc.) nerves and motor (movement) nerves. Many procedures may require the surgeon to handle or even cut nerves, which may cause changes in the senses or in movement. These are usually temporary. Most commonly though, a postoperative change in sensation results from the use of a numbing anesthetic that was injected close to the surgical site. If the local anesthetic works as the surgeon intends it to, it will block pain signals to the brain for as little as hours to as many as one to two days, depending on the type of local anesthetic used.

Pain and soreness

A certain level of pain will be present after any surgery. It can be hard to quantify in advance because of the variability between patients, the unpredictability of nervous-system reactions, and the different perceptions of pain that patients can have. Doctors expect that patients will call the level of pain soreness. This soreness can be considerable, especially if the surgery involves handling or moving muscles. Severe, uncontrollable, acute pain can signal a problem, such as infection or bleeding, and the surgeon should be notified immediately.

Frequently, a patient needs prescription narcotics after surgery. It should be possible to transition to over-the-counter acetaminophen (Tylenol) after the first few days to weeks. Acetaminophen does not affect clotting.

Medications that inhibit clotting should be avoided both immediately before and immediately after surgery. These include anti-inflammatory medications, such as aspirin, ibuprofen, Aleve, Motrin, Advil, Mobic, and the COX-2 inhibitors (Celebrex, Bextra, and Vioxx).

Nausea/vomiting

After surgery, patients frequently suffer from nausea and even vomiting. There are several reasons for these discomforts. Many anesthetic agents have the potential for nausea or vomiting as a side effect. Narcotics and sedatives cause the stomach and digestive tract to slow down and may cause food or gas to build up in the stomach. The body may be placed in an unnatural position during and after surgery, affecting digestion. Patients may be uncomfortable due to side effects of antibiotics or pain medications. The nausea should resolve over the first twelve to twenty-four hours. If not or there is acute pain in the abdomen, the patient should contact the surgeon.

Constipation

Constipation occurs frequently after surgery. As with nausea, constipation can occur because of the use of sedative drugs, disruption of the normal eating routine, and side effects of pain medications. Especially if the patient has a history of constipation, stool softeners should be used after surgery, but they should be stopped if antibiotic drugs cause diarrhea.

Frequent urination

In the first six to twelve hours, the fluids given to a patient during surgery may cause a patient to need to urinate frequently and with more volume than usual. During the next few days of recovery, this increased urination may persist if body fluids caused by the inflammation and healing processes need to be excreted. Frequent urination should not raise concerns unless there is also painful or bloody urination. In fact, having less urine than usual is much more worrisome than having more than usual (see below).

Sore throat or cough

General anesthesia involves the placement of a tube in the throat and the use of gases that cause irritation or inflammation of the throat and lungs. Therefore, it is common to have mild sore throat or cough after surgery.

Potential problems

These postoperative problems should cause a patient to notify the surgeon's office as soon as possible.

Fluid collection or excessive drainage

While some drainage from a closed surgical wound can be expected, large amounts of fluid coming from a wound can be an important thing to tell the surgeon. Many procedures require the surgeon to move a large number of body tissues, which leads to the buildup of fluid from inflammation. First, inflammation delivers extra fluid and cells to promote healing. Second, swelling (edema) can occur when normal fluid drainage (through lymph vessels) is disrupted. The extra fluids that accumulate after surgery may be able to escape the body only through the wound itself, causing excessive drainage.

Surgeries with the potential to cause significant fluid buildup are well-known to plastic surgeons, and a drain may be used to eliminate these fluids. However, there are problems with drainage if there is an unusual fluid buildup or when fluids are not adequately drained due to malfunction or another reason. This may lead to a fluid collection called a seroma, which is at increased risk of infection. The fluid may develop a tract to the incision and drain significantly.

Drainage may rush out of the body or flow continuously via the drain or the incision. The fluid is usually yellow to clear, but in the first six to twelve hours, the fluid may appear pink. A very small amount of blood can turn the fluid pink or even a light red. Bandages and dressings that are excessively or continually saturated with this pink or light-red fluid do not indicate an emergency, but the patient should notify if drainage seems excessive in volume.

Bleeding and hematoma

It is worrisome if there is drainage of colors other than clear, yellow, pink, or light red. Bright-red drainage may indicate ongoing bleeding. Deep-red or black drainage may indicate a hematoma. A hematoma is an enlarging collection of blood, which is quite worrisome and should be reported because it may require exploratory surgery and is associated with infection, skin death, and other complications of uncontrolled bleeding.

Infection

The typical signs of infection are fever, redness, swelling, and pain. Unfortunately, these are all expected events after surgery as well. Fever is very common in the first few days after surgery, especially low-grade fever in the 99–101 degree range. This is due to inflammation of the surgical site and the lungs from surgery. Temperatures higher than 101 or persistent for several days should be reported after inspecting for the other signs of infection. Redness is a sign of inflammation, which occurs with surgery, but if an infection is present, the redness would be more severe and tends to enlarge in size and become brighter red over time. Asymmetric or significant swelling or pain should be reported. White, thick, or foul-smelling drainage also suggests that there is an infected wound and that it requires early treatment.

Constrictive dressings

Dressings are of course common after surgery and are applied with care and based on expected swelling. Instructions may state to not remove dressings, but bandages and dressings can be too tight if swelling is more than expected. There is more potential for this complication with dressings that wrap around an extremity, especially if that extremity is not elevated above the heart. In an extremity, areas farther from the heart than the surgical site will have excessive swelling. A dressing that is too tight may compress and block blood flow, causing pain and swelling and, ultimately, the death of tissues. If these symptoms develop, the surgical team should be notified and the dressings loosened.

Neurologic effects

Some patients can experience altered levels of alertness, headache, decreased energy, impaired vision, or other nervous-system effects after surgery. Minor symptoms can be monitored and should improve, but deterioration or significant changes should be reported.

Heart and circulatory-system effects

Surgery is a stressful event, and there are many effects on the body. While cosmetic surgery is generally reserved for healthy patients, it should not be assumed that all symptoms after surgery are normal. Symptoms of problems with the heart and blood vessels, such as chest pain, shortness of breath, fast or irregular heartbeat, or an acutely swollen or painful leg should be reported or treated via 9-1-1 or emergency room.

Inability to urinate or insufficient urination

Surgery, anesthetic agents, and swelling may impair the production of excretion of urine. If the patient is making urine but is unable to urinate, pain and pressure will build up in the lower abdomen. Urinary retention, as this is called, may require drainage with a catheter if it does not resolve on its own. This is more common in men due to enlargement of the prostate. A small amount of urine output may indicate urinary retention or may mean that the body is not making enough urine for a more serious reason, such as dehydration or kidney malfunction, and needs evaluation.

Skin Aging and Damage

The Structure of Skin

The skin is the largest organ of the body. It is the protective barrier between the external environment and the individual, so it has many roles regulating temperature, regulating metabolism, preventing infection, slowing down an excessive loss of water, and reflecting and absorbing ultraviolet radiation. Because it is the most visible organ, the skin readily shows the relentless changes caused by aging and exposure to the environment.

The skin is composed of two major layers: the epidermis on the outside and the dermis just beneath. Fatty subcutaneous tissue lies below the dermis (see figure 1).

Figure 1. Layers of the skin: epidermis and dermis

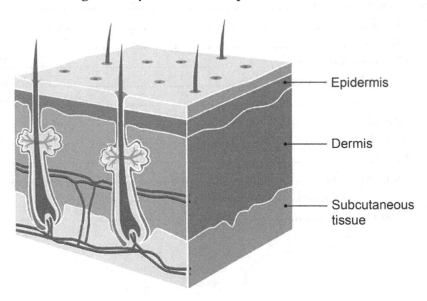

Functional Problems

Dry Skin

Dry skin will feel rough, scaly, itchy, and wrinkled. Primarily caused by loss of water through the stratum corneum of the skin, dry skin is especially troublesome in dry climates and during the dry winter season. As individuals age, the stratum corneum becomes even less resistant to water evaporation, so drying of the skin occurs more often. Bathing actually aggravates dry skin, and skin does better with quick baths or showers and quick towel drying. Antibacterial soaps and liquid soaps are extremely drying. Bland, uncolored, unperfumed soaps are preferable. Oils and moisturizers should be applied after drying: Soaking in bath oil only prolongs exposure to the drying water. Humidifiers are beneficial and should be used to increase humidity during dry weather and in heated rooms.

Oily Skin

Oily skin results from increased secretion of natural oils and sebum, which should be considered a helpful, natural lubricant. Oily skin is smoother, less wrinkled, and better protected from sun damage. Excessive oiliness, however, may result in clogged pores that cause an increased propensity for acne.

People with excessively oily skin should not scrub with abrasive facial products, which may actually stimulate more oil secretion by sebaceous glands. Rather, it is better to cleanse with a mild soap and avoid soaps containing rich emollients from vegetable, mineral, or silicone oils. Astringents, which contain mostly alcohol, may improve oiliness initially, but they are irritating, can cause the skin to flake and peel, and should be used infrequently and cautiously. Individuals with very oily skin do not need lotions or moisturizers. If the skin is mildly oily or becomes dry from use of astringents, oil-free moisturizers or oil-in-water mixtures should be used.

Combination Skin

Some individuals have a combination of oily and dry skin. The oily skin most commonly occurs on the nose, chin, and forehead, while the cheeks are often dry. In this situation, it is again important to avoid abrasive peels and astringents. If there is a significant difference between the skin types in each region, treatment should moisturize the dry areas, and cautiously apply astringents to oily areas. If the differences between the areas are slight, patients may use cleansers for combination skin and avoid using moisturizers.

Behavioral Effects on Skin

Facial Exercise

Despite significant marketing, there is no scientific evidence to confirm that facial exercises make any difference in preventing or reversing facial aging due to wrinkling or the effects of gravity over time. Maintaining good nutrition is more valuable to beauty of the skin.

Nutrition

A healthful, balanced diet is essential for all organ functions, and the skin is no exception. Malnutrition causes a myriad of whole-body illnesses that also affect the skin. Even well-nourished individuals can improve their well-being and the skin's luster with a healthful diet. A healthy diet will provide the necessary calories, vitamins, previtamins, and minerals. (Natural processes in the body can turn previtamins into the vitamins it can use.) If an individual eats a diet that is deficient in the fat-soluble vitamins—A, D, E, and K—disease can occur. This is also true of the water-soluble vitamins, B complex and C. The B-complex vitamins include folic acid, riboflavin, niacin, thiamine, pyridoxine, and cyanocobalamin.

High-fat diets can lead to inflammation and hardening of the arteries (atherosclerosis) and cancer. Saturated fats specifically contribute to aging and cancer. Individuals should also be well hydrated to encourage normal function of cells. Dehydration prevents normal moisturizing of the skin, but overhydration will not moisturize the skin. A skin-healthy diet includes plenty of whole grains, fresh fruits, vegetables, olive oil, and fish oil. Antioxidants are important because they scavenge and remove oxygen free radicals. These may be applied topically to the skin (vitamins A, C, E, and selenium) or taken by mouth (vitamins A, C, E, and coenzyme Q10).

Smoking

Smoking causes the skin to develop a dehydrated stratum corneum that has thicker elastin and fewer blood vessels. The skin of a smoker is drier, coarser, thicker, and more wrinkled. Smoking disrupts the skin's microvasculature (the density and number of tiny blood vessels), impairing blood supply to the skin. Smoking also creates oxygen free radicals, which accelerate wrinkles, photoaging, and skin cancers. These problems are also discussed elsewhere.

Stress

Stress can lead to hives and acne breakouts in acne-prone individuals. Chronic stress and muscle tension can cause excessive frowning and muscle activity with associated frown lines and furrows.

Sun Exposure

The sun is the focal point around which our world revolves. We all need some exposure to feel well. Sunlight is also important for the production of vitamin D. However, the sun's ultraviolet (UV) rays also cause the most damage to our skin. Most of this damage is done during youth, by the age of twenty years. The sun's radiation is made up of different wavelengths of light: about 2.5% to 3% are ultraviolet. The rays have an intermediate wavelength that is slightly shorter than that of the violet rays of the visible light spectrum. There are three wavelengths of UV light, called UVA, UVB, and UVC:

- UVA light penetrates deeply into the dermis, damaging the skin's collagen and elastin fibers. It does not cause a burn, but it does stimulate melanin production, which produces the suntan. Long-term exposure causes photoaging and skin cancer by producing oxidants that damage the DNA of skin cells.
- UVB light causes sunburn. Inflammation causes the redness seen after acute exposure. UVB also contributes to DNA damage and photoaging.
- UVC is filtered out by the ozone layer of Earth. It would be destructive to skin if it were to pass through the ozone layer. As the ozone layer depletes, UVC is of much greater health concern than before.

A suntan is the skin's defense against UVA rays. Chronic exposure to these rays causes melanocytes to produce irregular patches of melanin: freckling, brown spots and splotches, and hyperpigmentation. The skin also becomes wrinkled, rough, and leathery and has a dull complexion, age spots, and spider veins (telangiectasia).

Tanning beds, if properly calibrated and maintained, primarily deliver UVA rays, resulting in a tan but not UVB rays, which cause burns. Chronic exposure to tanning beds is very damaging to skin because UVA rays produce oxidants, which damage DNA.

Sunblocks and Sunscreens

Both sunblocks and sunscreens help protect skin from UV exposure. Sunscreens work either by blocking sunrays or by absorbing rays. Traditionally, sunblocks were inorganic compounds (zinc oxide and titanium oxide), whereas sunscreens were organic formulas (listed below). However, sun products usually now have a combination of agents. Sunscreens are graded by their sun protection factor (SPF), which measures protection against UVB rays. The SPF multiplies the amount of time you can spend in the sun without being burned. For example, if a sun exposure would cause you to burn in ½ hour with no sunscreen, then a screen with an SPF of 4 would allow you 2 hours' exposure before sunburning occurred. An SPF of 15 would therefore provide 7½ hours of protection. Apply sunscreen liberally and frequently, usually every half hour and after swimming or exercising.

It is important to select a screen that blocks or absorbs both UVA and UVB rays. You must check the product's ingredients against the list below. Knowing SPF alone is not adequate since it tells you nothing about UVA protection.

- ❖ Sunscreens are organic compounds that block UVA or UVB rays or both:
  - ➢ Blocks UVB rays only
    - Cinnamates such as octyl methoxycinnamate
    - Homosalate
    - Octocrylene
    - Octyl salicylate (octisalate)
    - Oxybenzone and methoxybenzone
    - PABA (Para-aminobenzoic acid)
  - ➢ Blocks UVA rays only
    - Avobenzone

> Blocks UVA and UVB rays
  - Anthranilates
  - Benzophenone-3
  - Oxybenzone
❖ Sunblocks are inorganic compounds that protect against both UVA and UVB rays. Products with a high percentage (>5%) of the following are most recommended by medical professionals.
> Titanium oxide
> Zinc oxide

Conclusions

Skin serves many important functions in protecting the body. It also shows the signs of aging that people cannot see in other organs. With proper care, as discussed in the next chapter, these signs can be minimized and occasionally reversed. Ultimately though, treatments that are more aggressive are usually necessary and are discussed later in this book.

Skin Care and Rejuvenation

Skin-Care Products

The skin-care industry is a maze of marketing. Labels make many claims and promises, but only an educated consumer can sort out the truth. It is important to read the ingredient list on each product. Possible claims include the following:

- ❖ *Antiaging.* There are no antiaging creams. The only substances that will inhibit the environmental damage are sunscreens and sunblocks.
- ❖ *Natural product.* There may be naturally occurring ingredients in the product, but there are usually many additives, including preservatives, fragrances, dyes, and other chemicals.
- ❖ *Hypoallergenic.* Any substance may stimulate a reaction if a person is allergic to that substance. Most reactions to products, however, are not true allergic reactions but rather irritations due to chemical sensitivity. One frequent allergy is to the sunscreen PABA, but this is rarely used anymore for this reason.

Soaps

Soaps come in liquid or bar form: liquid soaps are milder. The surfactants in soap may be drying to the skin if they remove too much of the oil (sebum) from the skin surface. Likewise, soap can leave the skin feeling oily if not enough sebum is removed.

Synthetic soap is an alkaline substance with a pH of up to 10. (A neutral pH is 7, a pH less than 7 is acidic, and a pH greater than 7 is alkaline). Skin, on the other hand, is slightly acidic and has a pH of 5 to 6. Synthetic soaps may be drying and irritating to the skin. Natural soaps contain nonalkaline materials and tend to be less harsh than synthetic soaps because of their lower pH. These soaps are commonly made from avocado or citrus juices. If a particular soap, natural or synthetic, is causing irritation, soap with a lower pH may help. Most beauty soaps are synthetic with a lower pH and may be labeled "pH-balanced." They are, ideally, less drying and may have a moisturizing additive.

Some soaps, known as superfatted soaps, are less drying because of the addition of fatty additives, such as cocoa butter, lanolin, or petroleum. These soaps make the skin oilier. Transparent soaps are made with fats and glycerin; they tend to be less harsh. Soap may cause irritation due to fragrance, color, or preservative additives. Deodorant soaps contain antimicrobial agents, which can be irritating in some individuals. Chemically sensitive individuals should choose uncolored and unscented soaps.

Toners

Toners are solutions or lotions containing water, alcohol, and other ingredients such as salicylic acid, propylene glycol, and witch hazel. Toners are meant to remove impurities, cleansers, superficial skin cells, oils, and soap residues. They may be beneficial for oily skin by removing excess oil, and they may be beneficial to dry skin by removing the excess stratum corneum of epidermis. Unfortunately, they can also be very irritating to the skin, so users should have a limited trial before adding toners to a regular regimen.

Moisturizers

Dry skin is caused by evaporation of water from and through the skin; the more evaporation, the drier the skin is. Each individual has a genetic predisposition to water loss. As people age and skin is damaged by the sun, the stratum corneum is less able to block evaporation. Greater water loss is also seen in a drier environment. A moisturizer applies a film on the skin that reduces water evaporation. It helps most individuals, but if a person already has oily skin, it can clog pores and aggravate acne.

Oil-Based Moisturizers

Oil-based moisturizers derive their function from emollients. These emollients may be derived from mineral oil, petrolatum, silicone, animal fat, sheep wool (lanolin), fish oil, vegetable oils, vitamin E, or some combination of these. Emollients occupy the spaces between keratinocytes, smoothing and lubricating rough skin. Oil-based moisturizers leave a film but last longer. Eucerin is an example of an oil-based cream.

Oil-Free Moisturizers

Oil-free moisturizers are water-based creams. They are preferable for those with oily or acne-prone skin, are easier to apply, and do not leave much residue. However, the duration may be limited, and significant humidity is necessary for them to work. Most creams and lotions on the market are water-based.

Most oil-free moisturizers generally contain the following substances, called humectants:

- Glycerin or propylene glycol, which attract and bind water from the environment to rehydrate the skin
- Lactic or hyaluronic acids, which are naturally occurring skin molecules that bind with water to provide a protective film on the skin

Antioxidants

Antioxidants are a class of molecules that block and absorb the oxygen free radicals produced by normal metabolism. Free radicals are unstable, high-energy molecules known to cause damage to DNA and cellular proteins, so they are an important cause in the aging process. Antioxidants such as selenium and vitamins A, C, and E are very important components of one's diet. Preliminary research suggests that antioxidants play a positive role in inhibiting cancer and heart disease. However, the role of antioxidants in topical products and cosmetics is currently unknown: there is little evidence suggesting that antioxidant additives penetrate the skin below.

Exfoliants

As mentioned before, skin cells form in the base of the epidermis and migrate to the surface over several weeks to become part of the stratum corneum. The cells are then shed. They can, however—and especially in older skin—stick and clump in the stratum corneum, causing a delay in shedding. Pores become clogged and sebum can build up, resulting in acne-prone skin. The lack of shedding causes skin to appear cracked, causing a dull, flaky, irregular skin surface.

Exfoliants are designed to remove these excess cells from the stratum corneum. When effective, they leave the skin looking smoother and shinier. Exfoliating products that physically remove dead skin are quite common. Facial masks are effective but irritating and drying to most people. Abrasive sponges disrupt and absorb oils but can be very irritating to many skin types. Hydrocolloids, or water-based exfoliants, can be difficult to control. Mudpacks may be effective in oily, acne-prone skin. Vinyl rubber works by sticking to the oils on the skin surface then holding the oil and clumped skin upon removal. Products that chemically remove dead skin are alpha hydroxy acids, beta hydroxy acids, and tretinoins. Their mechanism differs from that of many common exfoliants, which physically remove debris and skin cells. Patients need to understand that routine use of any exfoliating agent is relatively recent and long-term effects are still poorly understood.

Alpha Hydroxy Acids (AHAs)

Treatment with alpha hydroxy acid gives the skin a smoother, fresher look. AHAs penetrate the superficial stratum corneum and break cells apart to help shed dead skin. The disruption of connecting bonds between cells is essentially the result of a superficial burn; the depth of activity depends on the concentration of the acid. They cause tingling and redness, which subside quickly when weaker concentrations are used. However, it will not eradicate wrinkles, clogged pores, or acne.

These water-soluble solutions are either natural extracts from various plants or fruits or synthetic products from the laboratory. Common acids include the following:

- Citric acid, found in citrus fruits and pineapple
- Glycolic acid, found in sugar cane juice, sugar beets, or grape juice
- Lactic acid, found in tomato juice and milk
- Malic acid, found in apples or pears
- Tartaric acid, found in grapes and wine

Glycolic and lactic acids are commonly used because of their excellent skin penetration. Initially, as the cells shed from the stratum corneum, the skin becomes flaky. It generally will smooth within ten to fourteen days. The different acids will have different effects on various skin types, so inflammatory responses can vary from negligible to extensive redness.

The activity or strength of a solution depends on two factors: acidity (pH) and concentration. Products with pH of less than 3 are too acidic and irritating, while those with a pH of greater than 5 are usually inadequate and achieve very little. The active ingredient in AHA products ranges in concentration from 1% to 15%. Mild solutions contain 4%–7%, while stronger preparations contain 8%–15% concentrations. Clearly, with higher concentrations, there are more problems with irritation. Most people do not tolerate long-term use of concentrations greater than 15%.

In conclusion, it is preferable to start conservatively with alpha hydroxy acids with a 7%–8% concentration that have a pH between 3 and 5. They should be used once daily, preferably at night. Then if there is no problem, twice-a-day treatments are recommended.

After using AHA exfoliants, it is imperative to use a sunscreen during the day if one is outside or in the car because the outer, protective layer of skin has been removed and the natural ultraviolet barrier is significantly weakened. Generally, maximum benefits are noted within 6 to 12 months. Then a maintenance regimen is used to maintain skin improvement even with reduced frequency of use or concentration of the product.

Beta Hydroxy Acids (BHAs)

Beta hydroxy acids are in a relatively new class of exfoliants. Currently available beta hydroxy acids are best used in the 1%–2% strength with a pH of 3 to 4. Like AHAs, they function by disrupting skin-cell bonds, encouraging shedding. The difference is that beta hydroxy acids are oil-soluble, while alpha hydroxy acids are water-soluble. This allows sebum (skin oils) and pores to be deeply penetrated and disrupted, improving the care of oily skin.

BHA solutions include salicylic acid, benzoic acid, butyric acid, and willow-bark derivative. Salicylic acid is the main ingredient in aspirin, and it seems to provide many of aspirin's anti-inflammatory properties, limiting redness and irritation. Symptoms of irritation may still include redness, burning, itching, pain, and possibly scarring. People with darker-colored skin are at a higher risk of scarring and pigment changes. As with alpha hydroxy acids, protection from sun exposure after use is very important.

Tretinoin

Tretinoin is a drug that is synthetically manufactured from vitamin A. All product versions require a doctor's prescription. Brand-name products include Retin-A, Renova, and Activa. Currently Retin-A and Activa are approved by the United States Food and Drug Administration as acne drugs, while Renova is approved for treatment of both acne and sun-damaged skin. All three drugs, however, are generally prescribed for acne, sun damage, and the treatment of fine wrinkles.

The greatest changes occur in the first six months and include a thinner, smoother stratum corneum, larger cells that are more evenly hydrated, a thicker epidermis with a more even pigmentation, fewer wrinkles, more blood vessels, and evidence of increased collagen formation. The skin appears smoother with improvement in color and fewer irregularities, such as freckles, brown spots, and hyperpigmentation. Tretinoins are not effective for erasing deeper wrinkles or correcting damaged skin.

Tretinoins are agents that work by breaking the bonds between skin cells in the stratum corneum. Thus, cells are shed more easily and pores are unplugged. Tretinoins may be applied as a solution, cream, or gel in increasing concentrations of 0.025%, 0.050% and 0.100%. It is preferable to start with lower or medium concentrations, using them once daily at night. As irritation subsides, concentrations may be increased. After initial use, the skin may be red, dry, flaky, or peeling. A daytime moisturizer or weak steroid cream (1% hydrocortisone) may help with irritation. Due to increased sensitivity to sunlight, using effective sunscreens is essential.

After six months of use, tretinoin use is reduced to a maintenance regimen with a lower frequency or concentration.

Bleaching Agents

Bleaching agents are used to downregulate the production of pigment that has led to hyperpigmentation. This hyperpigmentation may be due to genetics, inflammation, or sun damage. The most common bleaching agent is hydroquinone, which is used topically to inhibit the production of melanin at a DNA level. Kojic acid reduces the enzymatic activity producing melanin. Niacin decreases the delivery of melanin. Retinoids like tretinoin also decrease the production of melanin and enhances the effects of those above.

DNA Repair and Growth Factors

Although much of the above agents are designed to alter or correct problems after they have occurred, it is also possible to provide enzymes that protect the DNA from the damage caused by stressors such as UV light, free radicals, and smoking. In addition, growth factors can provide the proteins and stimulation necessary for cells to be able to renew themselves during the cell-turnover process.

Laser Types and Technology

The acronym LASER stands for light amplification by stimulated emission of radiation. Lasers are classified by the wavelength (or color) of light they produce and by the source of the light. The skin naturally contains compounds like melanin that give skin its different colors. Lasers of different wavelengths target these compounds, selectively dissolve them, and cause relatively minimal collateral damage to surrounding skin.

Laser light is produced in either continuous or pulsed waves. The light can also be modified to use a higher power with a very short-pulse duration, as in the Q-switched lasers.

Type of Laser	Tanning	Wavelength (nm)	Responsive lesions
Pulsed lasers			
Flash lamp-pumped organic dye (vascular)	Yellow	577,585	Vascular lesions
Flash lamp-pumped organic dye (pigmented)	Green	510	Pigmented lesions
Copper vapor	Green	511	Superficial pigmented lesions
Copper vapor	Yellow	578	Vascular lesions
Continuous-wave laser			
CO_2	Invisible (infrared)	10,600	Excision or vaporization of multiple lesions
Nd:YAG	Invisible (infrared)	1064	Vascular and pigmented lesions
Argon	Blue-green	488 - 514	Vascular lesions
Krypton	Green	521, 530	Pigmented lesions
Krypton	Yellow	568	Vascular lesions
Q-switched lasers			
Ruby	Red	694	Pigmented lesions, tattoos
Alexandrite	Red	755	Pigmented lesions, tattoos
Nd:YAG (frequency doubled)	Green	532	Pigmented lesions, tattoos, vascular lesions

Figure 2. Lasers will be discussed throughout this book in various sections, but the following table summarizes their general uses.

VASCULAR LESIONS
(RELATED TO BLOOD VESSELS)

Angiomas

Angiomas, more specifically cherry angiomas, are red, blood-filled lesions a few millimeters in size that can become larger and raised over time. These benign tumors of vessels that develop with age are not usually associated with any underlying disease and are of cosmetic concern only. They do not regress on their own. They can be treated with electrocautery, radiofrequency ablation, cryotherapy, or laser therapy, preferably pulsed dye laser with the goal being complete destruction and healing with slight scarring without expected recurrence of that lesion but expected progression of others.

Hemangiomas

Infantile hemangiomas are similar to cherry angiomas in that they are tumors of vessels but they form in infancy and tend to regress over time. They may become quite large and can damage the overlying skin in the process. Treatment is urgent in situations with frequent bleeding, ulceration, obstruction of vision or breathing, or if causing heart failure due to high flow rates. Treatment is also beneficial in keeping the nonacute hemangioma from becoming as large and to encourage regression earlier. Treatments used are steroid injections, pulsed dye laser therapy, and beta blockers (a type of blood pressure medication). Surgery may be necessary for the collateral damage done to skin and soft tissues.

Port-Wine Stains

These are capillary malformations that are present at birth but become progressive with age. They begin flat and pink but become darker, thicker, and larger through the decades, ultimately causing irreversible damage to overlying skin. They cannot be cured but can be curbed with pulsed dye laser therapy, which sequentially damages the feeding blood vessels while trying to protect the skin.

Venous Lake

Venous lakes are dilated nests of small veins (venules) that occur later in age due to damage to the lining of the vessels due to sun damage, which allows dilation of the vessels. These can be excised or controlled with laser, electrical, or radiofrequency destruction.

Rosacea

Rosacea presents as redness of the nose, cheek, chin, and forehead. Flares occur with triggers: exercise, sun, wind, temperature swings, stress, alcohol, or spicy food. Subsequent development of small pumps with pus (pustules) and thick, bumpy skin is expected. Rosacea can be curbed with suppressive antibiotics, skin care, phototherapy (IPL), and pulsed dye lasers.

Spider Veins

The cause of spider veins (sunburst varicosities or telangiectasias) is poorly understood, but it is thought to be the effect of circulating estrogens. Other contributing factors include weight changes, prolonged standing, and genetic predisposition. These typically form in the lower extremities first. This is, as expected, largely due to gravity. The veins in the lower extremities have valves that, when functioning, propel blood back to the heart against gravity when the leg muscles contract. However, as these valves wear out, increased back pressure builds up, leading to dilation or enlargement of these vessels. There is a higher incidence of spider veins in women than in men, probably because of the vessels' greater exposure to estrogen.

Telangiectasias appear as simple linear vessels, multiple branching vessels, or tiny vessels radiating in a spider shape from a central point (the reticular vessel; see figure 3). Spider veins are true blood vessels that carry blood, which are not to be confused with the larger and darker blood vessels called varicose veins. They do connect superficial veins to the deep veins of the legs, but they are not essential and can be destroyed.

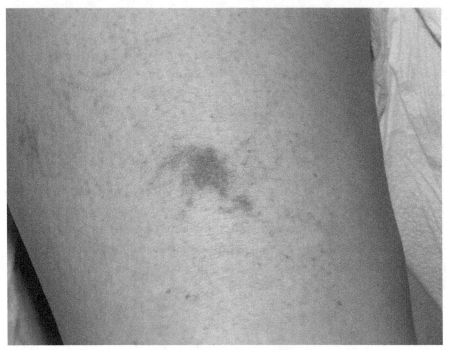

Figure 3. Photograph of spider veins (telangiectasias), borrowed from WFUBMC Plastic Surgery

The minimally invasive forms of treatment for spider veins are electrodesiccation, sclerotherapy, and lasers.

Electrodesiccation

In electrodesiccation, a tiny needle is inserted into the vessel, and an electric charge coagulates the vessel. The vessel and trapped blood are then slowly reabsorbed. The canals often reform and the vessels reappear, requiring repeated treatments.

Sclerotherapy

Tiny amounts of a chemical that hardens blood vessels, called a sclerosing agent, can be injected into a vessel to force it to harden; later, the body will absorb the trapped blood and vessel wall.

Fortunate patients may see significant improvement after two to three treatments; however, it is not unusual for patients to require eight to ten treatments. Once the spider veins are adequately controlled, the individual may need to return periodically for maintenance injections. Depending on the area treated, cost varies from $150 to $750 per session. A session will usually last from 20 to 30 minutes with injection of up to 6 cc of solution. This will treat most areas on both legs.

Technique

Substances that are commonly used in this therapy include hypertonic saline (a very concentrated saltwater solution), sodium tetradecyl sulfate, and polidocanol. When the substance is injected into the vessels, an immediate flush will be noted as the agent flows through these tiny vessels. The vessel will reappear only to be absorbed over a period of weeks. The procedure may be uncomfortable, with a burning sensation at each area injected. Ice applied to an injected area minimizes the burning sensation.

Recovery

Some physicians like to wrap the legs after a session or apply compression hoses for two to three weeks, although this is generally not necessary beyond a few days. Injections can be repeated safely at six-week intervals. Complications are rare, but they include ulceration and scarring if the solution is injected into surrounding tissues rather than into the vessel. On occasion, individuals may develop hyperpigmentation of the injected spider area, but this usually resolves within several months.

Lasers

Lasers targeting the wavelengths of hemoglobin, a major component of blood, can treat telangiectasia with relative sparing of the skin. Depth of penetration is controlled by wavelength: Longer wavelengths of light mean deeper penetration. Longer pulse durations are used to treat larger vessels.

Lasers used in the treatment of telangiectasias include Nd:YAG (1064 nm) for deeper vessels, long-pulsed alexandrite (755 nm) or diode (800 nm) for vessels in the reticular dermis, and PDL (585 nm) for superficial vessels. The pain is variable with different lasers but can be controlled through various methods.

Varicose Veins

Patients with spider veins often have associated problems with varicose veins. Varicose veins are larger and deeper and are characterized by dark, bulging vessels. Valves in the leg veins help keep blood moving toward the heart: Varicose veins result from an incompetence of these valves in veins that connect the superficial skin veins with the larger veins deep in the leg. Varicose veins are common after multiple pregnancies and in individuals who spend a lot of time on their feet. They are also a natural consequence of aging. These veins may be painful and associated with recurrent swelling (see figure 4).

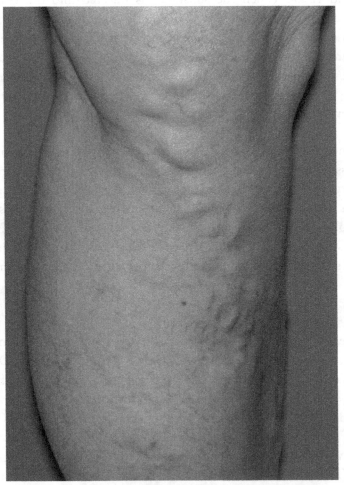

Figure 4. Photograph of varicose veins. Borrowed from WFUBMC Plastic Surgery.

Patients with varicose veins need to be evaluated for deep vein blockages before any type of treatment is given. This can be accomplished by Doppler flow studies, noninvasive ultrasound testing that illustrates blood flow in the veins. Varicose veins are significantly more difficult and complicated to treat than spider veins.

Isolated varicose veins may be amenable to sclerotherapy. After an injection treatment of true varicose veins, most surgeons apply a compression wrap for forty-eight to seventy-two hours. Patients who have varicose veins treated with sclerotherapy have a much higher incidence of dark-skin pigmentation after treatment.

Large or extensive, true varicose veins are best treated by surgically removing the vessels or by ablating them with radiofrequency. Radiofrequency is typically delivered via a catheter inserted into the veins and coagulating the vein as it is pulled through the vein.

HAIR CARE

Although it serves no discernible function in human beings, hair imparts social and sexual connotations. It provides important attributes to the feminine mystique while reflecting youth and masculinity in men.

Hair follicles are skin appendages. They provide the materials in hair and everything needed for growth and development of its roots. The follicle is a living structure, well nourished by a rich blood supply, whose health determines the continued viability and growth of hair. Hair follicles are distributed over the entire body, except on the palms of the hands and the soles of the feet.

The activity of hair follicles is perpetually dynamic. There are three phases in a follicle's life. On the scalp, hair growth proceeds at a rate of 0.3 mm per day, and each hair grows for several years; this is the growth phase called anagen. Then the follicle spends several weeks in the catagen phase, during which time the base of the hair moves toward the skin surface. The hair is shed during the final resting (telogen) phase, which also lasts several weeks. Then the process begins anew. In the scalp, about 85% of the follicles are growing hair in the active phase (anagen), 1% is in catagen, and 14% is resting in telogen. Scalp hair grows more rapidly in women than men, while the reverse is true of body hair. Normal scalp loses about 100 hairs daily. The anagen phase is shortened to only six months in the eyebrows, axilla (armpit), trunk, and extremities. Catagen and telogen have the same duration. This explains the limited length of eyebrows and the reason they do not require haircuts.

Between 90,000 and 140,000 hairs are present on a healthy scalp. Generally, the thicker the shaft, the less dense the scalp hair will be. Individuals with thick, dark hair actually have fewer hair follicles than those with thin, fair hair.

Hair variations characterize different ethnic groups: East Asian hair tends to be thick and straight on cross-section, with vertically oriented, straight follicles. Hair of African origin has curved follicles that are often parallel to the skin surface in places, producing tightly coiled, curly hair. Caucasian hair follicles tend to be elliptical and slender.

Hair may be defined as dry or oily and coarse or fine. Hair follicles are surrounded by sebaceous glands. As individuals with fine hair have thinner hair shafts, there is room for more sebaceous glands. Accordingly, those with fine hair have oilier hair than those with coarse hair do. Variability in hair oiliness is determined by genetic predisposition and by hormonal balance. Women often note an increase in hair oiliness during their menstrual cycles. The gender differences in facial, pubic, and other body hair—except eyebrows and eyelashes—are determined by different sex hormones.

The newborn infant characteristically demonstrates a fine down of hair, described as vellus hair, which covers various parts of the body. As the infant ages, vellus hairs at several specific sites, such as the scalp, develop into the pigmented, thick hairs called true or terminal hair.

Hair Care

Hair care influences the quality, texture, and durability of hair.

Shampoo

All shampoos leave small amounts of buildup behind on the hair after rinsing. Some shampoos coat the hair shaft, making the hair look dirty and unmanageable. Over time, the accumulated buildup from a shampoo reduces that shampoo's cleaning effectiveness. Changing shampoos helps remove the previous shampoo's buildup and restores the hair's natural beauty. Changing shampoos frequently is therefore a good part of healthy hair care.

Detergent shampoos remove too much sebum and dry the hair. Even very oily hair may be dried excessively by detergent shampoo. Dry, brittle hair should be shampooed less frequently and is best washed once, not twice, at each shampooing. Hydrating shampoos absorb water and aid in swelling the hair shaft, thereby producing a thicker appearance.

Conditioners

Conditioners make hair shiny and more manageable, counteracting the drying effect of shampoo and reducing the hairs' static adherence. Various hair types respond differently to any particular conditioner. Choosing the ideal conditioner may require trial and error before a specific selection is made. Always avoid conditioners that leave a heavy coating on the hair.

Gels, Mousses, and Sprays

Gels and mousses will moisten and thicken hair by binding themselves within the hair shafts. Some products contain silicone, which tends to make the hair smoother, calmer, softer, and more manageable. Avoid products, such as sprays, that contain alcohol. These tend to make the hair dryer and more brittle.

Permanent and Body Waves

Permanent waves make hair curlier and wavier by making the hairs thicker. The procedures need to be repeated every three or four months, and they may damage the hair because of the chemicals they use. Good hairdressers should pay attention to the response of an individual's hair to these treatments.

Coloring

Hair-coloring products contain many chemicals that may cause damage to your hair. It is essential to choose a careful, experienced, attentive hairdresser who can minimize potential damage. Individuals with thinning hair will find that dark-hair coloring makes hair look even thinner because it contrasts with the underlying scalp. Just as this contrast between dark hair and light scalp aggravates the appearance of thinning, lightening the hair color and leaving light or gray hair untouched disguises thinning hair.

Styling

A good hairstylist should be able to camouflage balding areas by using appropriate styling. Thinning hair is magnified by long hair; the heaviest hairs tend to separate from the others, revealing the underlying scalp. Layering the hair and keeping it short can create an illusion of a thicker head of hair.

Dandruff (Seborrheic Dermatitis)

Dandruff is the most common cause of scaling of the scalp. The yellowish scaling most commonly affects the back and sides of the scalp.

It is not caused by a dry scalp, so adding oily solutions is not the correct treatment. Antidandruff shampoos should be used with great care: although they usually correct the problem, they may not be good for the hair. A good alternative approach is to use the usual shampoo, then clean, massage, and apply antidandruff lotion once or twice weekly.

Cosmetic procedures can move, restore, and remove hair more easily than ever before. A plastic and reconstructive surgeon can be a patient's first resource in hair concerns and will be discussed in the next chapters.

Hair Loss and its Treatment

Causes of Hair Loss

Hair loss (alopecia) as a consequence of aging occurs in 20% of women and 70% of men. The degree of loss ranges from significant thinning of scalp hair to varying patterns of baldness.

Male and Female Pattern Baldness

Male and female pattern baldness are known medically as androgenetic hair loss. The signs of male pattern baldness commence after puberty and during early adolescence. By age 40, hair thinning becomes evident both in the hairline at the forehead and on the crown of the head. Hair on the back and sides of the scalp is typically spared (see figure 5). There are seven patterns of male baldness that are well depicted by Norwood's classification.

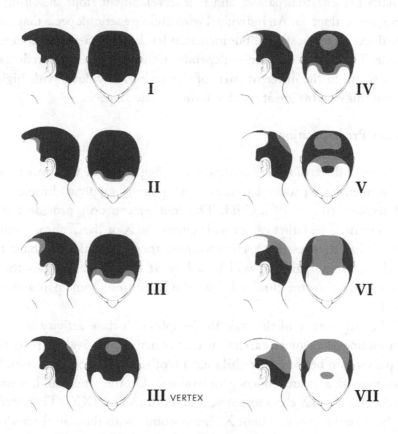

Figure 5. Photographs of Norwood's classification

Hormonal Factors

Testosterone is the masculinizing hormone; estrogen and progesterone are the predominant feminizing hormones. Both sexes are vulnerable to hair loss. Female hair loss may become evident during menopause and, occasionally, after pregnancy, when the protective influence of estrogen may be lost. Hormonal imbalance from the use of birth-control pills may also cause hair loss.

An enzyme called 5-alpha reductase causes some men to lose their terminal (true) hair in androgenetic hair loss. It causes the terminal scalp hairs to revert to the barely visible vellus hairs by converting testosterone to dihydrotestosterone. This new hormone thins hair shafts by attaching to hair follicles and preventing the normal blood supply to reach the follicles, producing progressively finer hairs with each new growth cycle. Eventually the hairs become transparent, and hair development stops, resulting in androgenetic alopecia. An individual with androgenetic alopecia may have normal levels of testosterone but increased levels of the 5-alpha reductase enzyme. The pattern of baldness depends on the level of 5-alpha reductase that is found in the different parts of the scalp. Individuals with higher levels of this enzyme are at risk for androgenetic alopecia.

Genetic Predisposition

A short discussion of hereditary can help explain why more men than women have pattern baldness. Both parents supply a chromosome to determine the sex of a child. The mother can only provide the X chromosome. The father can provide either the X or the Y chromosome. If the father supplies the Y chromosome, then the child will have the XY chromosome pair and will be a boy. If the father supplies the X chromosome, then the child will have the XX chromosome pair and will be a girl.

The only source of the trait for 5-alpha reductase activity is the X chromosome. If a woman carries the trait of activity for 5-alpha reductase and passes it to her son, that child has no other X chromosome from his father to mask a future tendency for baldness. On the other hand, women and girls have two X chromosomes, from both parents (XX). Therefore, a daughter would have to inherit X chromosomes with the trait for 5-alpha reductase activity from both parents to develop female-pattern baldness.

Many assume that the hair status of a man's maternal grandfather may indicate future hair loss patterns, but there are many more genetic factors that determine the age of onset, pattern, and extent of hair loss.

Scalp Infection or Trauma

Any traumatic injury or burn extensive enough to injure the deep layers of the dermis can permanently destroy hair follicles, causing hair loss in the affected area. Similar scarring alopecia can be seen with skin diseases such as discoid lupus, lichen planus, scleroderma, and tinea capitis (ringworm).

Infection

Fungal or bacterial skin infections involving the scalp may result in hair loss. The degree of scalp involvement may range from mild redness and irritation to affliction with open sores. Proper medical attention, correct diagnosis, and appropriate medications will usually cure the underlying condition. However, scars in the scalp may damage hair follicles and limit or prevent future hair growth.

Traction Alopecia

Any physical force, or traction, that continuously pulls on the hair may lead to permanent hair loss. This may be observed in people who use hair-replacement systems. These include hair weaves, braids that incorporate synthetic hair, or a hairpiece that has been bonded or glued to the existing hairs. Similarly, tight braiding may cause hair loss. Treatment involves reduction or elimination of the traction. Hair loss may become permanent if it continues for a prolonged period of time.

Trichotillomania

Trichotillomania is an anxiety condition in which a person compulsively and repetitively twirls and pulls on his or her hair. Over time, there may be enough injury to the underlying hair follicles to convert the temporary, self-induced hair loss to permanent areas of baldness. Treatment involves counseling and possibly antidepressants.

Systemic Illness

Constitutional or Emotional Stress

Occasionally, the stress of a serious systemic infection, pregnancy, emotional trauma, or surgery may precipitate a sudden, total loss of hair. In this process, known as telogen effluvium, follicles prematurely exit the active growth phase and enter the resting phase. The hairs are typically shed two to three months after such an event. Fortunately, regrowth of hair usually occurs after the event that caused it is resolved.

Hair loss may be associated with severe metabolic and nutritional disorders, just as it may occur in individuals who are seriously ill. Hair loss does not occur as a pure consequence of a badly balanced diet or vitamin deficiency.

Endocrine System Disorder

Hair follicles are sensitive to many hormones that are produced in excess. Reversible hair loss may be seen in hyperthyroidism or in hypothyroidism, as well as diabetes mellitus. Excessive production of hormones from the pituitary gland and adrenal cortex may cause scalp hair loss. Unfortunately, it may also cause women to experience excessive hair growth and hair growth in locations where only men typically grow hair (a condition called hirsutism).

Autoimmune Disorder

Although the exact cause of alopecia areata is unknown, it is thought to be an autoimmune process in which antibodies attack a person's own hair follicles. This causes distinct patches of hair loss with no other symptoms. Normal regrowth of hair occurs within four to six months. The process may, occasionally, involve the entire scalp and cause complete loss of hair upon the head (alopecia totalis) or loss of all body hair (alopecia universalis). Alopecia areata affects nearly 1% of the population at some point in life.

No treatment cures alopecia areata, but symptomatic treatment is available. Topical steroids and injections of steroids into the bald area help hasten the regrowth of hair. Minoxidil (Rogaine) and tretinoin (Retin-A) have been used to promote hair growth and will be discussed later. Severe cases may be treated with oral steroids or immunosuppressants, but these carry significant side effects.

Drug Therapy

Drug treatments for many illnesses can cause hair loss. Listed here are some of these drugs and examples of their uses:

- Lithium treats depression.
- Amphetamines are used for narcolepsy, depression, and ADHD.
- Warfarin (Coumadin) and heparin are used as anticoagulants (blood thinners).
- Oral contraceptive pills prevent pregnancy.
- Propylthiouracil treats hyperthyroidism.
- Allopurinol treats gout.
- Gemfibrozil lowers cholesterol.
- Chemotherapeutic agents treat cancer.
- Radiation therapy treats cancer and other illnesses.

Both chemotherapy and radiation therapy initiate a process known as anagen effluvium. Unlike in telogen effluvium caused by stress, hair loss is sudden because hair does not enter a resting state before being shed. In some patients, all hair may be lost; in others, only the 85% of hair that is in the active phase during treatment may be lost. Hair growth usually returns after treatment.

Cosmetic Aids

Usually the first step for patients wishing to treat thinning hair or alopecia is to use camouflage products. These products do not treat the underlying condition but, instead, aim to hide them. There are several camouflage products available for those who wish to create the illusion of a fuller head of hair. Invisible concealments are available at most cosmetic stores. These may be applied to the scalp to reduce contrast with the hair color.

- DermMatch is sold as hard-packed colored powders that create an illusion of much thicker hair. To apply properly, it is massaged by fingers into the scalp at sites of thinning hair. It shades areas without hair and coats existing hairs, making them appear thicker.

- Couvré lotion delivers micronized organic proteins directly into the hair, thickening the shaft and creating an illusion of thicker hair. It is available in several shades.
- Hair-building fibers contain keratin fibers that bind to hair fibers, making hair look thicker. Examples include the Great Cover Up, Organin, Nanogen, and Toppik.

Hairpieces

Manufactured hairpieces can be added to existing hair. Today's hair addition systems are significantly better than in the past. They can provide an aesthetic, comfortable, and practical solution for most circumstances.

The hairpieces may be constructed from donated human hair or from synthetic fibers. While human hair has the advantage of color match, flexibility of styling and coloring, and authenticity, it is usually heavy and more expensive ($1,000). Human hair works better with longer additions. Pieces made of synthetic fiber are lighter and less expensive ($50 to $150) but have a likelihood of color fading and look less natural because of their difficulty blending with the wearer's own hair.

The modern manufacture of hairpieces is far removed from that of the old wig with its heavy fabric base. A natural appearance can be achieved with a well-constructed, well-cut, and well-combed piece using hair that matches the recipient's own hair color. However, using too much hair and creates an unnatural look. One should choose a hair addition system that is light, comfortable, natural-looking, and easy to maintain. Potential drawbacks of hairpieces include an unnatural hairline and part, displacement when swimming or in the wind, discomfort when hot and sweaty, and the need for frequent maintenance or replacement.

One must carefully research all alternatives and the reputation of the hair addition center being considered. The American Hair Loss Council in Chicago, Illinois (www.ahlc.org), is a good place to start the research.

Hairpiece Attachment

Modern hairpieces typically use a light, nylon mesh base with glue to adhere to the scalp. Some wearers prefer a strong, durable base that is molded to the scalp using pressure from the fingers and applied with double-sided tape at several points on the base. Other options include hair weave, bonding, or integration. Techniques that sew the hairpiece to the scalp have been abandoned because of the frequent occurrence of scalp infection and scarring.

Hair Weave

With hair weaves, residual natural hair along the sides and back of the scalp is braided and intertwined to attach the hairpiece base. The front of the hairpiece still attaches to the scalp with double-sided tape. Monthly rebraiding and reattachment is necessary, and traction baldness may develop over time. The piece is often unduly bulky where it overlaps the braided hair, but its attachment is secure under windy conditions or during contact sports.

Bonding (Fusion)

Cyanoacrylates create rapidly drying glue that provides a natural appearance when used on a hairpiece whose base is made of plastic and a light mesh. The head may be shaved completely to provide full attachment; alternatively, a piece can be custom-fit to a bald area, and natural hair may be combed in with it. As with the hair weave, monthly reattachment with appropriate servicing of the piece is necessary. Traction alopecia may occur, causing further loss of natural hair. Exertion and sweating may cause the glue to melt, permitting the piece to become loose and displaced. Swimming, with its exposure of the bonding product to chlorinated water, may also weaken the attachment of the hairpiece.

Hair Integration

Integration is an excellent technique for those who have significant thinning without obvious, large bald areas. A weblike addition is created with natural or synthetic hair. The individual's remaining hair is brought through the webs, blending with the natural hair and holding the addition in position.

Medical Treatment of Hair Loss

Minoxidil (Rogaine)

The FDA approved minoxidil (Rogaine) to reduce high blood pressure, although it was originally tested as an oral antacid. Researchers discovered that, after several weeks of treatment for high blood pressure, oral minoxidil promoted the growth of new vellus hairs. Unfortunately, fewer than 5% of patients taking oral minoxidil to treat hair loss will respond with dense growth of scalp hair.

Topical Rogaine has been available as a nonprescription lotion in 2% and 5% concentrations for several years. It has to be applied twice daily for a prolonged period of time for any growth to occur. In the first four months, fewer than 5% of patients using topical minoxidil will respond with a perception of dense scalp hair growth, while 20% of patients will develop a minimal amount of new vellus scalp hair. At one year, 40% of patients showed a response. Topical minoxidil is best used for men under forty years of age and who began balding recently, within the last five to ten years. Areas of baldness on the vertex of the scalp (top of the head), rather than on the temples, respond most favorably by growing new hair. An excellent regrowth of hair is not seen very commonly.

Minoxidil dilates blood vessels—that is, it is a vasodilator—it increases blood supply to hair follicles. Another hypothesis is that it prolongs the growth cycle of hair follicles. And another is an increase in growth factors at the base of the hair follicle in response to topical minoxidil. Despite the unclear mechanism, the result of minoxidil treatment is hair that is longer, thicker, and less likely to fall out in some patients. It is probably more effective in preventing baldness than in reversing hair loss. When topical application of minoxidil ceases, progressive hair loss resumes and the extent of baldness becomes apparent within several months.

The disadvantages of minoxidil are a requisite long-term commitment, its high cost ($50–$90 per month)—it is not covered by health insurance, and its side effects include itching, headaches, near syncope (swooning), and occasional heartbeat irregularities. Because it is a vasodilator, it is not recommended for anyone with heart disease or who is over age 49. Its long-term safety remains unknown.

The response rate in women with thinning hair who apply topical Rogaine appears to be superior to results in men: hair becomes longer and thicker. It is best used in thinning hair and works best on the frontal scalp in women.

Tretinoin (Retin-A)

Although tretinoin (Retin-A) has been tried in men and women with hair loss, there is no convincing evidence of its efficacy for this condition. It does appear to enhance the effects of minoxidil.

Hormonal Manipulation in Men

Certain drugs known as 5-alpha reductase inhibitors (Propecia, Proscar, and Avodart) block the conversion of testosterone (the masculinizing hormone) into dihydrotestosterone, which causes the hair-loss syndrome, as discussed previously. Some current evidence exists that these drugs are an effective remedy for hair loss. Finasteride is a first-generation 5-alpha reductase inhibitor, marketed as Propecia for hair loss. It is also known as Proscar for treating noncancerous overgrowth of the prostate gland. A second-generation inhibitor, dutasteride, is available for benign prostatic hypertrophy under the trade name Avodart. By reducing the amount of dihydrotestosterone in the body, androgenetic alopecia is reduced.

Side effects of the 5-alpha reductase inhibitors include male breast enlargement (gynecomastia) and reduced libido (sexual drive). These products are not approved for use in women, children, or men considering conception of a child: It is harmful to the fetus. They are expensive ($60 per month), and hair loss recurs after use is discontinued.

Hormonal Manipulation in Women

Estrogen replacement after menopause has not demonstrated any appreciable improvement in hair regrowth in women, nor have scalp injections of cortisone or progesterone been helpful in this regard.

Hair-Replacement Surgery

Surgical correction of hair loss has become a routine part of cosmetic surgery. It provides a dynamic process of hair replacement.

Hair Transplantation by Graft

As opposed to the common perception of transplantation as use of tissue from another individual, hair transplantation means taking hair as a graft from a donor site on the patient's own scalp (back or sides) and moving it to areas of baldness. Hair loss leading to baldness typically involves the hairline at the forehead and may extend upward into the frontoparietal scalp and the vertex frontoparietal occipital scalp. The band of hair around the sides (temporal areas) and back (occipital areas) of the scalp usually survives for the patient's lifetime. Therefore, moving hair from these areas to the area of baldness will survive for the rest of the patient's life. It will continue to grow at the normal rate of ½ inch per month because growth behavior of the donor site is dominant.

Transplantation is not recommended for individuals whose total baldness leaves fine, silky hair on the back and sides of the scalp. A well-constructed, customized hairpiece better serves them.

Variations in the transplant regime may be varied by factors such as age, extent of the baldness, color and thickness of hair, and the extent of the donor area. Ethnic differences can be important. The hair in African Americans tends to come straight out of the scalp, while in Caucasians, it comes out more at an angle. Afro-Americans also are more prone to keloid scarring, and a careful review of their scar history is necessary.

There are several types of grafts used depending on the shape and size of the tissue transplanted. The overwhelming trend now is to transplant follicular unit grafts. This kind of graft is as a small piece of tissue containing fat, hair follicle, and hair (graft). The following are the actual dimensions of graft units: 4 mm (punch graft), 3 mm (punch recipient), 1 mm (micrograft), 5 mm (narrow strip graft), 8 mm (wide strip graft), and 2 mm (slit graft).

Illustrations of different grafts and their dimensions are shown in figures 6–8.

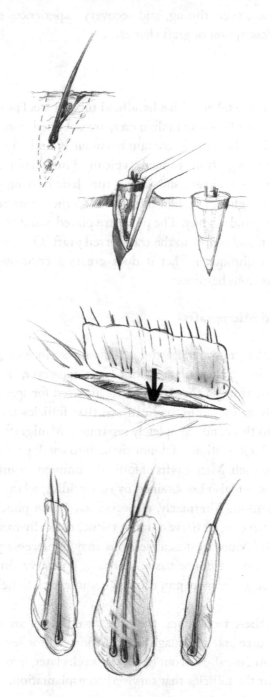

**Figures 6, 7, 8. Illustration of graft techniques: (A)
punch grafts, (B) slit grafts, (C) micrografts**

The surgeries, their timing, and recovery experiences are discussed below, after a description of graft shapes.

Punch Grafts

Punch grafts are taken with a handheld tubular steel punch. Multiple round "plugs," typically 4 mm in diameter, are obtained from hair-bearing areas of the scalp. These grafts contain between 10 and 15 hairs per plug.

A smaller punch graft instrument, typically 3 mm in diameter, removes bald plugs from the recipient site. The 4 mm hair-bearing grafts, which tend to contract slightly, are then transferred to the 3 mm recipient sites, which tend to expand slightly. The plugs are placed about $1/_8$ inch apart to allow adequate blood supply to the transferred graft. One of the problems with the plug technique is that it does create a cornrow appearance, especially at the front hairline.

Minigrafts and Micrografts

These smaller grafts reduce the patchy appearance of punch grafts; further, donor sites are usually not noticeable. However, the grafted area may appear quite thin, so these tiny grafts are used for specialized needs. Looking closely at the scalp, one can see that follicles are clustered in groups of two to three, not completely separated. Minigrafts are obtained by subdividing large sections of donor tissue into small grafts that contain three to six hairs each. Micrografts of follicular units containing a mere two to three follicles can also be obtained by subdividing a larger donor graft under magnification. Alternately, a specialized 1 mm punch instrument or an injection needle can harvest donor tissue, typically from the back or side of the scalp. More treatment sessions may be necessary because the increased dissection of donor tissue increases operative time. The extra time makes these grafts more prone to loss because each follicle experiences increased trauma.

In each of these techniques, the transferred plugs are typically held in place with gauze and a bandage around the head for several days. The transplanted hairs usually fall out about six weeks later, and a new growth phase begins for the follicles that survived transplantation.

Strip Grafts

Strip grafts, which are also taken from the back and sides of the scalp, consist of long segments of hair-bearing skin between 5 mm and 8 mm wide. Each strip contains as many as 35 hairs. The strips are harvested with a scalpel and then transferred to slit incisions made in the recipient site. The graft is placed pointing in the direction of adjacent hair and is fixed in position with sutures. It is preferable to take narrow strips because wide strips create a skin incision that is often too taut in the donor area. This technique is most frequently used to create a new frontal hairline that is then combined with punch grafts on the remainder of the scalp.

Slit Graft

Slit grafts are similar to the strip grafts, but they are much smaller. Each graft contains up to about ten hairs. The shape of these grafts may be hexagonal, square, or rectangular. Strip and slit grafts were developed to avoid the corn-row appearance caused by plug grafts, but they can result in an unnatural, tuft-like appearance.

Surgery Timelines, Principles, and Recovery

In most instances, a combination of the above techniques will be necessary at various stages to achieve the desired result. The hair-transplantation procedure requires multiple surgical sessions, depending on the size of the bald area and the fullness of hair desired by the patient. One should count on an interval of between two and three months between surgical sessions. It can take up to two years to obtain the final result. These procedures are typically quite expensive. Usually one to four serial treatments are necessary, at a cost of $3,000 to $10,000 per treatment.

Oftentimes, plugs and strips are used initially, while mini- and micrografts are used at subsequent sessions to fill in any intervening spaces. These can be combined with single-hair transplants to reconstruct a natural-looking hairline. Regardless of the type of graft used, the graft will be positioned to grow in the same direction as natural hair.

Hair transplantation is done with local anesthesia and occasionally with sedation. The amount of time for the procedure depends on the specific technique and the amount that the patient and doctor think can be achieved at any given session. Some doctors who transplant multiple, single-hair grafts prefer lengthy procedures of up to eight hours, referred to as mega-sessions. During each procedure, the donor sites in the back or side of the head are individually closed with stitches, or the entire donor area is excised, and the incision edges are brought together, leaving a single straight scar hidden by the surrounding hair.

Postoperatively, mild to moderate discomfort is easily controlled with medication. Patients should be able to return to work or light activity in several days. Physical activity can be advanced carefully, and patients should be back to most activities within several weeks.

As with all surgical procedures, there are risks of complications.

- *Bleeding.* Although rare, there may be bleeding at either the recipient or donor site. This usually can be controlled by holding pressure over the oozing wound. If there is continued bleeding, the surgeon may need to control it.
- *Infection.* Infection is rare. Any redness or drainage around the recipient or donor site may require local incision care and antibiotics.

The most likely problem is not a surgical complication but rather a disappointing result. A patient may be disappointed by the creation of an unnatural hairline caused by a cornrow appearance, an exceedingly low hairline, or a cobblestone appearance. If the hair transplants are not carefully placed, hair will grow in an unnatural direction. If grafts are not harvested skillfully, the hair follicles can be injured, causing minimal regrowth of hair.

Scalp Reduction

Scalp reduction (galeaplasty), is ideally suited for individuals with baldness involving the back and top of the scalp. If frontal baldness is also present, it must be corrected with hair transplants or other means. Scalp reduction procedures cost $1,500 to $3,000, depending on the extent of the procedure and the type of anesthesia necessary.

Technique

In scalp reduction, a portion of the bald area is excised, and the scalp surrounding the removed area is lifted, brought together, and closed with sutures. The amount of bald area that can be removed depends on the amount and looseness of the adjacent scalp. Several different patterns may be used to excise the bald area based on the shape of the bald area: a simple ellipse surrounding the bald area for smaller areas, a lazy S or a Y in the center of the bald area to make the scar less obvious, or if the entire bald area cannot be removed, it can be reduced with a J taken along one side of the bald area or a U along the entire edge of the bald area.

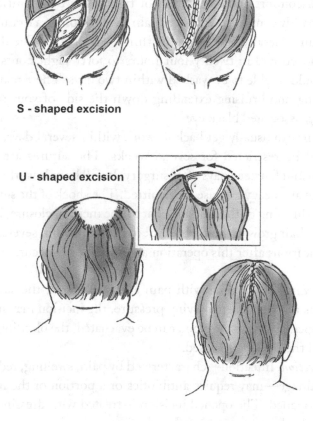

S - shaped excision

U - shaped excision

Figure 9. Illustration of scalp reduction incisions

73

As with hair transplants, scalp reduction can be performed as outpatient surgery with local anesthetic and possible sedation. After excision of the bald area, the incision is directly closed with sutures. The wider the segment of bald scalp removed must be, the more loosening, or undermining, is needed on the adjacent scalp. If a very wide area has been taken, it may be necessary to lift and move the scalp down to the level of the ears on each side. Even these large scalp reductions or scalp lifts can be done under local anesthesia, but your doctor may recommend heavy intravenous sedation or even general anesthesia in some circumstances.

Recovery and Complications

A dressing may be applied. On occasion, if a large area has been removed and the incision is bloody, a suction drain may be placed to remove any accumulating blood or fluid. The scalp may have mild to moderate discomfort and a sensation of tightness. Any significant pain should be readily controlled with oral pain medication. If a drain has been placed, it can generally be removed within a day or two. The dressing is usually removed within twenty-four hours to forty-eight hours, and the incision should be able to be washed within two days. There may be some mild swelling and bruising extending down the side of your scalp and, occasionally, associated black eyes.

A patient can usually get back to work within several days, although activity will be restricted for several weeks. The sutures are removed between ten and fourteen days after surgery. It will be at least three or four weeks before any heavy exercise is permitted. The shock of the surgery may cause some thinning of the hair adjacent to the incision closure, but this is limited, and hair growth should be back to normal within several months.

Complications after this operation are rare but can occur:

- *Bleeding.* If bleeding with pain and swelling at the surgical site does not stop after applying pressure, the incision may need to be reopened so that the blood can be evacuated, the bleeding stopped, and the incision reclosed.
- *Infection.* Infection—characterized by pain, swelling, redness, and drainage—may require antibiotics or a portion of the incision to be opened. The opened incision is treated with dressing changes until it heals or can be reclosed.

- *Scar.* The scar is usually well hidden by hair, but if it widens, there will be an area of baldness. On the other hand, any hairs that fall out next to the scar will usually regrow in several months.
- *Stretch-back.* The biggest problem with the scalp reduction procedure is stretch-back, a widening of the scar and loss of some of the correction of the bald area. The risk for stretch-back can be minimized by designing the surgical excision very carefully and limiting excisions to seven to eight centimeters. A subsequent scalp reduction may be needed to correct stretch-back. Another alternative is limited hair transplantation into the area of stretch-back. However, hair transplants are less successful in scar bed tissue.

A second scalp reduction may be part of the original plan or, as mentioned, may be needed to correct stretch-back. In either case, the second procedure will be done after enough time has elapsed for adequate healing, regrowth of blood vessels to the operative site, and loosening of the adjacent scalp. Most doctors like to wait about three months before proceeding with another procedure.

Scalp Flap Transfers

A scalp flap is a portion of tissue that is excised and moved to another area but kept attached at the base to maintain a blood supply. Flaps of hair-bearing scalp can be moved to areas of baldness. The advantage of flaps is that a large amount of hair-bearing scalp can be transferred to a bald area in one session, thus providing a quantity of hair that would require several transplant sessions to achieve. Scalp-flap transfers are larger procedures and typically cost more than scalp reduction or scalp expansion (see below). Procedures may cost $4,000–$8,000, especially when combined with touch-up hair grafts.

A flap's attachment to the scalp at one end will limit where the flap can be relocated. The scalp flap has to be very carefully designed according to the individual's available donor hair and the location and degree of baldness (see figure 10).

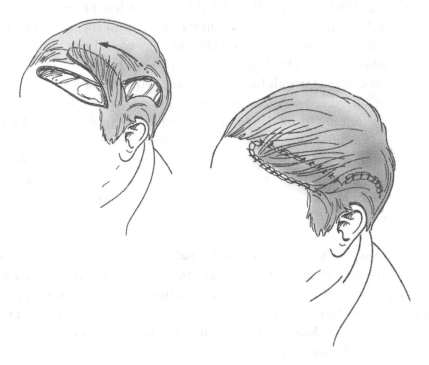

Figure 10. Illustrations of scalp flap

There are a number of different flaps:

- *Juri flap, also known as the temporo-parieto-occipital flap (named after Drs. Juri and Juri).* This is a long flap taken with its blood supply from the side of the scalp and extending around the back of the scalp. One such flap can reconstruct the entire frontal hairline.
- *Lateral scalp flap*: This flap is about an inch wide and extends along the side of the scalp. This flap will reconstruct half of the hairline, while a similar flap from the opposite side will reconstruct the other half of the hairline. Many doctors like to perform these two flap transfers at two separate sessions scheduled several weeks or months apart. The problem with both the Juri flap and the lateral scalp flap is that the hair coming from the flap will come out of the scalp in an unnatural backward slope. When using these two flaps, it is preferable to place them a little behind the hairline. Then in a subsequent procedure, the surgeon can reconstruct the hairline with a combination of micro- and single-hair grafts.

- *Temporo-vertical flap.* This is a vertical flap placed on the side of the scalp. It can be brought forward toward the frontal hairline and is advantageous in that it provides a natural direction of hair growth.
- *Occipito-parietal flap.* This flap from the side and back of the head can be used to correct baldness in the crown area.

Technique

As with the scalp reduction, scalp flaps can be performed as an outpatient procedure with local anesthesia for numbing and sedation for calming. The procedure will take several hours. The surgeon will trace and excise the planned flap. Once the surgeon determines exactly where the flap will lie, the matching area of bald scalp is removed, and the flap is sewn into place. These flaps carry their own blood supply with them, and generally, no hair loss occurs. At most, minimal, temporary hair loss occurs in the transferred flap.

Recovery and Complications

Oftentimes, suction drains will be placed to remove any blood and fluid that collect beneath the wound. These drains can be removed within one to several days. The incision may or may not have a dressing. If a dressing is used, most doctors will remove it within one to two days. There will be moderate pain with this operation, but it should be readily controlled with oral pain medication. Swelling and bruising around the operative site is common, but this resolves fairly quickly. Patients should be able to wash their hair within a couple of days. They will be out of work and limited in activity for at least five days; activity needs to be resumed slowly. Stitches are removed between ten days and two weeks.

Complications after this operation are rare but can occur. Most are the same as seen with scalp reduction and are not listed again here. Additional risks include the following:

- *Loss of hair.* Loss of hair is unusual after flap transfer. Temporary hair loss at the donor site is more likely if a wide flap has been taken and the incision is closed with too much tension. Too much tension on the incision closure can cause permanent hair loss in this area. It is imperative that tension is avoided.

- *Altered scalp sensation.* The flap may be numb; this numbness may be permanent if a larger sensory nerve is cut or injured. However, in most instances, sensation returns sufficiently so as not to cause a problem. There can also be temporary numbness at the donor area.
- *Abnormal direction of hair growth.* Hair may come out of the scalp in a backward position in some of these flaps. This can provide an unnatural appearance in the hairline. This problem usually can be camouflaged by subsequent transplants of mini-, micro-, or single-hair grafts.
- *Flap tissue death (necrosis).* This is the most feared complication of any flap surgery. If the flap that is transferred has inadequate blood supply, the flap—or more frequently, the tip of the flap—can die. Tissue death will require local incision care with dressing changes and possible surgical revision of the flap. If the flap cannot be readvanced to make up for the area lost, healing of the resulting open incision may take up to six weeks. Fortunately, this rare complication can be avoided with meticulous planning and skillful transfer of the scalp flap.

Scalp Expansion

Scalp expansion is an advanced form of scalp reduction and can be used in conjunction with scalp flaps. A balloon can be used to stretch the scalp just as large earrings can stretch earlobes and a growing fetus can stretch a woman's abdomen. This amazing ability of soft tissue to respond to pressure makes it possible to generate extra skin with hair to replace bald areas of scalp. A tissue expander in the form of a silicone-walled, inflatable balloon is surgically placed beneath hair-bearing scalp. This balloon device is attached to a valve located immediately beneath the skin. In the clinic, a needle is periodically inserted into this valve, and salt water (saline solution) is injected into the tissue expander. The tissue expander enlarges every time it is inflated.

As the tissue expander grows, it stretches the overlying hair-bearing scalp. Although the stretching process reduces the density of hair in the expanded scalp, the increased surface area of hair-bearing tissue more than compensates for the loss in hair density. As the expander gets larger, the overlying scalp will progressively bulge. Sometimes, two or more smaller expanders are more effective than one large expander. Once the scalp has been adequately stretched, it is prepared to replace an area of baldness by moving it during a scalp reduction or a scalp flap procedure. The increased surface area of the donor hair means that a larger amount of bald scalp can be removed without causing tension on the closure stitches. Decreased tension reduces the likelihood of the scar-widening or stretch-back complications, described previously in the scalp-reduction section.

While there are significant advantages to preexpansion of the donor scalp, there are obvious potential drawbacks. This procedure requires two operative procedures six to eight weeks apart and requires weekly visits for expander inflations. Once the expander starts to enlarge after two or three sessions, there will be a noticeable cosmetic deformity of the scalp. As the end of the expansion process is approached, significant distortion of the scalp will overlie the inflated expander. Further, because this strategy involves multiple procedures and an implant, the cost is usually higher than that for scalp reduction, typically $3,500 to $5,000.

Technique

Placement of the tissue expander can be done with local anesthesia as an outpatient procedure. The operation will generally take about $1^1/_2$ to 2 hours, depending on the number of tissue expanders placed. An incision is made at the junction of the bald area and anticipated scalp donor area. After placing the tissue expander, the incision is closed with sutures. There may or may not be a postsurgical dressing. The incision can be safely wet, and the hair can be washed within two days. The patient should be able to return to work after several days. The discomfort is mild to moderate and controllable with oral pain medication.

At the weekly doctor visits for inflation, the area will be cleaned, a needle inserted into the valve, and the implant inflated. This whole process only takes about five or six minutes. An uncomfortable feeling of scalp tightness can last for the remainder of the day of each expansion. Most of that sensation resolves within twenty-four hours. The operation for removal of the implant and reconstruction of the bald area is much as described in the sections on scalp reduction and scalp flap. Either strategy may be chosen for the second operation.

Recovery and Complications

Complications track those outlined in the sections on reduction and flap. The addition of a tissue expander after the first operation does add the potential risks and complications of the tissue expander. These include the following:

- *Infection.* An infection around the tissue expander will probably require the expander to be removed.
- *Extrusion.* On rare occasions, the expander will disrupt the stitches on the incision through which it was placed and become exposed. Depending on whether there is any infection, the expansion process may be continued despite the extrusion, or the expander may have to be replaced at that time or at a later date.
- *Implant leak.* In the unlikely event that the expander develops a leak, it will lose its saline solution and have to be replaced through a second operative procedure.

Conclusion

Once hair has been lost and a state of baldness is established, no currently available medication can restore cosmetically acceptable hair growth. Decisions regarding methods of hair replacement are clearly personal. Such a decision, however, will require a significant amount of research, including consultation with both cosmetology professionals who are knowledgeable about hair-replacement systems and skilled physicians who are familiar with all the techniques of surgical hair grafting and scalp reduction and transplantation.

If a patient has chosen a surgical solution, it is important to find an experienced surgeon who is competent in all areas of surgical hair replacement. The surgical procedure recommended should represent the best solution to the problem. It should not be proposed merely because it is the procedure with which a particular doctor is most comfortable. Costs are highly variable around the country for the various procedures. Full consultation should include a discussion of fees and expenses to be charged by the doctor and the facility, healing time and work time to be lost, and an honest discussion of potential risks and complications. This consultation should also make projections of the patient's future appearance: The doctor and patient must reach an understanding of a realistic, optimal cosmetic appearance and the amount of time it will take before the anticipated result is obtained.

HAIR REMOVAL

Hair Removal

Excess Hair

Some people seek hair replacement, but others increasingly seek cosmetic hair removal procedures. Some patients seek removal of undesired hair that is physiologically normal—it is a component of grooming for many people. Others seek removal of excessive hair.

Societal values determine the amount of hair that may adorn a woman's cheeks, upper lips, underarms, or legs. Ideals suggest that a woman should have no discernible hair at these sites, while males are expected to have only moderate body and extremity hair.

Several normal, natural causes of excessive hair growth include ethnic predilection (for example, women of Middle Eastern ancestry often manifest excessive facial and body hair); puberty, which causes hair growth in the pubic and armpit areas; and aging (after menopause, there is often an increase in facial hair growth).

Hirsutism, by definition, implies having too much hair; each individual will have a personal standard in this regard. Some women will develop excessive hair growth at sites that are normal for men, for example, on the face, chest, and ears. Such growth may occur without any clear, discernible, underlying cause and is called idiopathic hirsutism. Idiopathic hirsutism presumably results from an increase in sensitivity to, or excessive production of, androgenic hormones. No disease accounts for this simple growth of extra hair: the ovaries and menstrual cycles remain normal.

However, a person with excessive hair growth should see a doctor because this growth may have pathological causes—that is, disease. Appropriate clinical testing may be required to exclude diseases and other causes that are known to potentially lead to excessive hair growth. Examples include certain medications, tumors, and anorexia nervosa. Anorexia nervosa is an eating disorder that may lead to hormonal imbalance and excessive hair growth.

Three drugs or drug classes that are known to cause abnormal growth of hair are phenytoin (Dilantin), antihypertensive medicine, and cyclosporine. Phenytoin (Dilantin) is taken to prevent epileptic seizures. Antihypertensive medicine is taken to reduce blood pressure. Cyclosporine is an immune-modulating medicine taken to prevent organ transplant rejection.

Hormone-producing tumors of the adrenal glands or ovaries may lead to excessive androgen secretion and masculinization, including abnormal hair growth. The sudden or massive increase in hair growth that is typical of such tumors would cause most people to seek medical consultation rather quickly. A physical exam and laboratory studies will usually properly diagnose the underlying problem. The hair growth may be remedied by androgen-blocking medication or hair-removal techniques, but the tumor usually must be surgically removed.

Removing Unwanted Hair

Growth Inhibition

Some people wish to prevent growth of unwanted hair even as they remove hair they have. An important adjunct in hair removal is the topical prescription medication, eflornithine (Vaniqa). By inhibiting the enzyme ornithine decarboxylase, hair growth is impaired: It does not remove hair. It is approved only for use by women and should not be used by men or by women who are pregnant or nursing. It takes one to two months to take effect, and hair growth will resume one to two months after discontinuation. It is frequently used for thin, unpigmented facial hair that is difficult to remove with other methods.

Bleaching

Another technique to mask excessive hair growth is bleaching. This may be an acceptable method of making dark hair less conspicuous. It can be used over large areas of the body. Because irritation of the skin is possible, it would be wise to test for irritation by first applying the bleach to a small area as a patch test.

Waxing, Plucking, and Shaving

Hair may be physically removed with waxing. Cosmetologists sometimes use a wax technique to remove hair on the upper lip, chin, eyebrows, and legs. The heated wax is applied to the desired area. As it cools and sets, the wax is stripped off in the direction of the hair growth. Unfortunately, hair will regrow in a month. The procedure is painful and irritating to the skin. Infection of the follicles may develop. Isolated unsightly hairs can readily be plucked individually using fine tweezers. Both techniques are only temporary and also introduce the hazard of hair follicle infection. Equally temporary in its effect, shaving can mask excessive hair growth. Contrary to popular opinion, shaving does not increase the speed of hair regrowth, nor does it make hair coarser or darker. Pumice has been used successfully as an abrasive technique, but the process of hair removal in this manner is slow and tedious. It can also irritate the skin.

Depilatories

Excessive hair may be chemically removed with depilatories, which are chemical agents that dissolve hair proteins. One example is thioglycolic acid, which disrupts the chemical bonds called disulfide bonds that hold hair together. The irritation and minor breakdown of adjacent superficial skin occurs because skin cells also depend upon disulfide bonds: however, they are less targeted by thioglycolic acid because they contain lower percentage of the amino acid cysteine. To evaluate the skin's response and level of irritation, it is important to test this chemical on a small area before larger areas are treated. Topical steroids may ameliorate irritation. The depilatory may be applied as a foam, cream, or lotion to the appropriate areas and is allowed to remain at the hairy site for up to fifteen minutes before being removed. Depilatories are temporary because they affect existing hairs, not hair follicles. Depilatories may be used at home or in many settings, including salons, spas, and clinics. Costs are wide-ranging.

Electrolysis

A common permanent technique of hair removal is electrolysis. Electrolysis uses an electrical current to damage hair follicles. A fine needle is inserted into each follicle, and a burst of electric current destroys the hair root.

Although electrolytic therapy is meant to be permanent, regrowth of hair occurs 30% of the time, and treatment usually requires several treatments: It is not possible to treat the follicles in the telogen phase because of their lack of contact with the needle and their resistance. Treatment sessions are long, tedious, and expensive with a maximum of one hundred hairs being treated at a session. Treatments are mildly to moderately painful. Potential complications include hair return, altered pigmentation, infection, and scarring, including keloids. As with depilatories, electrolysis is performed in a wide array of settings, leading to inconsistency of costs to the patient.

Lasers

The most rapidly expanding area of hair removal is the use of lasers. Lasers propel pulses of light energy through the skin and target compounds that pigment the skin (usually melanin) within the hair follicle, thereby destroying any hair in the growth phase. Targeting skin pigments may not destroy all the targeted follicles at any one session, so repeat treatments at monthly intervals are required. Laser treatment is not a permanent method of hair removal, but it does target existing hairs and retard future hair growth. Again, it is better able to remove hair in the anagen (growth) phase and is more effective for darker hair. This is especially true for dark hair on light skin because there is much more melanin in the hair than in the skin.

The most common lasers used in hair removal are Nd:YAG, ruby, alexandrite, and diode. A laser works by converting light to heat energy, thereby creating a computer-controlled torch to cut, coagulate, and vaporize tissue. Its effect will be determined by power and time dosages to the area treated. Temporary redness and blistering may lead to local pigment changes. Local tingling or prickliness can be prevented by use of local anesthetic cream or cooling gels. Expertise in the use of laser machines is essential to reducing the potential complication of damaging tissue and causing scarring or hypopigmentation of skin.

Done properly, the technique can be effective, painless, and safe. Appropriate laser procedures are best performed under medical supervision even though laser hair removal is available at cosmetic laser spas. The patient must be informed of the risks and the potential benefits of laser treatment, as well as their duration, to provide maximal safety and desired effects and to detail the expenses involved. The cost depends on hair density, size, location, and type of treatment center. Cost ranges from several hundreds of dollars to thousands of dollars.

Conclusion

Hair removal is an elective cosmetic procedure motivated in some by a desire to remove unwanted, excessive hair and in others as a part of regular grooming. Sudden growth of excessive hair can signal side effects of drug-based treatment or even serious illness, so it should always be examined by a doctor. Lasers are the newest cosmetic procedures for hair removal; they join traditional methods and even chemical and electrical procedures in the modern arsenal against unwanted hair.

MINIMALLY INVASIVE FACIAL PROCEDURES

As skin ages, the deep layer of skin (dermis) becomes thinner, dryer, and less elastic, while the superficial layer (epidermis) becomes thicker and more clumped. Fine and coarse wrinkles develop, skin pigmentation changes, and the supply of blood vessels changes. Many of these changes are caused by exposure to sun, chemicals, wind, and gravity; further, the skin loses its ability to rejuvenate because genetic and physiological changes speed the process of aging. In addition, there are deeper changes that cause a loss of structures (fat, bone, cartilage, and muscle) that formerly supported the skin. Their disappearance contributes to the excess and flaccidity of skin.

These changes are represented by a thickening of the outermost layer of skin (stratum corneum) with clumped cells, abnormal cell growth that can lead to precancers or true cancers, degeneration of collagen and elastin fibers, a reduced number of proteins that hydrate the skin (glycosaminoglycans), and dilation of blood vessels into spider veins (telangiectasias).

The Face: Resurfacing the Skin

Skin resurfacing uses chemicals, manual dermabrasion, or laser light to desiccate (dry) or remove the outer layers of skin. Then, as skin regenerates from hair follicles and skin glands, it appears rejuvenated because the epidermis, dermis, collagen, elastin, and glycosaminoglycan proteins are more organized. This translates to reduced wrinkles, increased elasticity, improved hydration, removal of sun damage and precancerous changes, more regular pigmentation, improvements in scars, and reduced problems with inflammatory conditions of the skin (acne; seborrheic dermatitis; rosacea; and milia, which are small white cysts on the skin). Skin resurfacing cannot, however, correct the loss of structural support from muscle, bone, or fat. Loss of structure contributes to the signs of aging and creates deeper wrinkles and depressions.

The ideal candidate for skin resurfacing is a person of fair complexion with mild to moderate sun damage of skin that has adequate, deep structural support. Several factors make skin resurfacing a poor choice: darker-skin type, severe photoaging, pregnancy or breast-feeding, recent hair removal, a history of recent Accutane or radiation therapy to the area, a history of significant herpes outbreaks, and a history of hypertrophic (overgrown) scarring, or keloids.

	Appearance	Tanning
I	Pale, white skin / hazel eyes / blonde, red hair	Always burns, never tans
II	Fair skin / Blue eyes	Burns easily, poor tanning
III	Darker white skin	Burns prior to tanning
IV	Light brown skin	Mininal burning, tans easily
V	Brown skin	Rarely burns, readily tans
VI	Dark brown, black skin	Never burns, tans darkly

Figure 11. Fitzpatrick skin types

The risks of skin resurfacing are due to the controlled damage to important skin structures. If a patient has an unexpected response or if the resurfacing penetrates deeper than anticipated, scarring, pigmentation changes (loss of or excessive pigmentation), skin redness or sensitivity, or bacterial or viral infection can occur.

Chemical Peels

Chemical peels use a variety of chemicals to either burst or clump together skin cells, which lead to rapid exfoliation of either (1) the epidermis or (2) the epidermis with the superficial dermis beneath it. They are designed to treat signs of genetic aging and photoaging, including irregular pigmentation, reduced numbers of elastic fibers, fine wrinkling, and slow turnover of cells. The type of peel is classified by the depth of exfoliation as superficial, medium, or deep. The depth of peel chosen is determined by the patient's expectations, budget, and available recuperation time. Deeper peels work better at rejuvenating the skin but also prolong recuperation and increase risks of complications.

Chemical peels should be carried out by appropriately trained personnel. A superficial peel may be carried out by a technical assistant, while medium and deep peels should be performed by qualified health-care providers. Often, different areas of an individual's face require different peel depths to rejuvenate the skin. This technique requires the provider to have artistic ability.

The evaluation before the peel procedure must determine the degree of photo damage, depth of photo damage, changes to deep structures below the skin, and skin type. Darker-skin types (see table with Fitzpatrick scale, types IV–VI) may suffer significant skin-pigment alteration. Patients with a history of herpes at or around the mouth, recent Accutane, or abnormal scarring (with keloids) may not be good candidates for a medium or deep chemical peel, although prophylactic treatment can prevent a herpes outbreak.

After the procedure, a moist environment is preferred. With superficial peels, a moisturizer may be adequate. With medium and deep peels, this is usually obtained with an occlusive dressing or an emollient. Sun avoidance is essential until the skin has regenerated; sunscreen is important for several months after the procedure. The skin regenerates from skin appendages (hair follicles and skin glands), so areas with fewer appendages heal less predictably. Peels can be used even in areas that have fewer appendages than the face, but extreme care must be practiced in order to minimize complications. See table for a summary of chemical peels.

CHEMICAL PEEL DEPTHS

Superficial   Trichloracetic Acid (TCA)   30%
                  Jessners Solution
                  Salicylic acid ⎫
                  Lactate acid   ⎬ 14% each
                  Resourcinol
                  Alcohol

Medium   Trichloracetic Acid (TCA)   50%
             Jessner's Solution + TCA 35%
             Glycolic Acid + TCA 35%

Deep   Phenol/croton oil
           TCA 70%

Figure 12. Chemical peel depths and healing times

Superficial Peels: Glycolic Acid, Salicylic Acid, and Jessner's Solution

The most common alpha hydroxy acids (AHAs) are glycolic acid and lactic acid. These are the same acids used in exfoliation solutions, but they are applied in higher concentrations, typically between 20% and 70%. Salicylic acid is a beta hydroxy acid (BHA). Resorcinol is made synthetically from natural resins and can burst skin cells called keratinocytes. Jessner's solution is a mixture of resorcinol, lactic acid, and salicylic acid. These solutions disrupt ionic bonds between cells, and they are appropriate for a patient with fine wrinkles, mild lentigines or melasma, mild acne or acne scarring, actinic keratosis, ichthyosis (scaly skin), or xerosis (abnormally dry skin). There is a variety of proprietary peels with additional ingredients or strengths that can modify the efficacy of the peel for certain purposes.

A superficial peel is nonablative—that is, it does not remove the entire epidermis—but it removes the top two layers of the epidermis, including the horny layer). It stimulates healing and thickening of the epidermis and dermis. Glycosaminoglycans, skin proteins that attract water, are also increased after treatment, improving skin hydration. A superficial peel is appropriate for a patient who wishes to correct fine wrinkles and mild degrees of hyperpigmentation.

Technique

The skin is best pretreated with a two-week course of tretinoins or low concentrations of alpha hydroxy acids to smooth and cleanse the skin. The patient will lie down with the eyes protected. The face is cleansed to avoid pooling of acid and a blotchy result. The peeling solution, either a liquid or a gel, is applied and left on the face for several minutes. Then a neutralizing agent (water or bicarbonate) may need to be applied for several more minutes. The patient may feel mild stinging and itching.

Recovery

Negligible peeling may occur for a day or two, and a short-lived redness may show for three to five days, but the patient can resume normal activities immediately. Side effects are usually limited to irritation or dryness, but occasionally hyperpigmentation may be seen. Periodic, biweekly to monthly, treatments are best initially; they can be gradually spaced out.

Medium Peels: Trichloroacetic Acid (TCA)

Medium peels are ablative, so they remove the entire epidermis by reaching into the papillary (top layer of) dermis; occasionally, they reach beyond that layer into the deeper, reticular dermis. These peels remove areas of thickened skin lesions—such as calluses—while they tighten skin, reduce wrinkles, and fade hyperpigmentation. With the increased depth of peel comes significant additional improvements in skin elasticity, hydration, tone, and color, but also increased discomfort and risks of scarring, infection, and altered pigmentation.

Trichloroacetic acid (TCA) is the usual chemical used for the medium-peel depth. TCA causes keratin proteins to denature and coagulate (that is, deform and clump together), which causes the skin to subsequently scale off in layers. TCA can result in a superficial peel or a peel into the dermis, as is done with a deep peel or laser resurfacing (see below). TCA is often combined with other solutions such as Jessner's solution, retinoic acid, glycolic acid, or other proprietary mixtures, such as the Obagi TCA blue peel, which adds a visual blue color that allows the doctor to discern the depth of penetration.

Technique

Strength can be adjusted between 15% and 70% acidity to tailor to the appropriate depth of treatment. Depth of treatment is dependent on concentration and on preparation of skin; the number of applications needed during one session can be judged by the frosting that occurs during the procedure. TCA is neutralized by materials carried by the blood vessels of the dermis and, therefore, does not require provider neutralization. Pain is moderate during the procedure and may require sedation, but postprocedural pain is usually mild and rarely requires narcotics. Some swelling may occur. After the treatment, a moist environment is created with ointments, emollients, or tape.

Recovery

Peeling of epidermis and dermis may last for five to seven days, and redness typically lasts for seven to fourteen days. Cleansing can be done with soap or diluted hydrogen peroxide. Dermal healing continues for months, and improvement in the skin can occur throughout this time. Patients who develop hyperpigmentation because of inflammation should be treated aggressively with a bleaching agent. Hydroquinone is the most proven bleaching agent, but other alternatives are becoming popular as long-term use is associated with skin irritation and ochronosis, which is darkening of the skin. Most recommend that if using hydroquinone, it should be cycled with other bleaching agents such as kojic acid, arbutinin, azelaic acid, and others, especially in dark-skinned patients. Hydroquinone inhibits tyrosinase, which is important in the process of melanin production by the skin.

Deep Peels: Phenol

Deep peels or resurfacing lasers are indicated in patients with deeper wrinkles, moderate acne scarring, or severe melasma (brownish hyperpigmentation). Despite some claims, a deep peel will not lead to extreme tightening of the skin, remove pits and pores, or improve telangiectasias (dilated spider vessels lying in the deep layers of the skin). Deep chemical peels are ablative and remove the epidermis and upper dermis by extending into the deep layer of the dermis (the midreticular dermis). A deep peel leads to the deposition of new epidermis and dermis with at least partially renewed elastic fibers, glycosaminoglycans, and collagen. Deep peels have largely been replaced by lasers for the reasons cited below.

Risks

The deeper peels carry greater risks, especially in thin skin. If a peel is carried out too deeply into the dermis, it can result in scars. There also may be permanent color changes, which typically result in hypopigmentation, an enduring loss of the normal, pigmented color of the skin. Dark-skinned individuals may develop areas of hypopigmentation if they are sensitive to UV light and are not careful to avoid sun exposure in the early weeks after the peel. Significant herpes outbreaks and bacterial infections can occur without proper care.

Technique

The common deep peels are high strength TCA, i.e., 70% and phenol. Phenol is a coal tar derivative that is commonly applied with croton oil to achieve the deep peel. This is a deep, painful burn done only under sedation. The patient needs to be monitored and resuscitation equipment should be available. Phenol can and has resulted in serious cardiac arrhythmias when applied rapidly, so the physician must apply it slowly.

Recovery

After the deep peel, an occlusive dressing augments the depth of penetration of phenol. During the healing phase, the skin will be swollen and crusted, peeling lasts ten to fourteen days, and once the skin has healed, it will remain red for several months. Swelling can also be significant.

Dermabrasion

Dermabrasion is effective in improving deeper wrinkles and in improving the appearance of irregular scars by smoothing the face, much as a carpenter planes a board. It can be done on small areas to smooth scars or on the whole face to correct fine wrinkles or improve acne scars. The depth is controlled by the health-care provider and can span from superficial to full thickness. It is different from microdermabrasion, which is very superficial and can be performed by untrained personnel, even a patient at home. Patients with lighter skin colors are good candidates for dermabrasion, while the treatment of those with darker complexions (Asian skin and African American skin) can result in blotchy discoloration or hyperpigmentation.

Dermabrasion uses a rapidly rotating diamond burr or wire brush to sand the outer layers of skin. Microdermabrasion, on the other hand, uses propelled crystals or abrasion to exfoliate the epidermis, a technique that improves dilated pores, oily skin, and mild sun damage.

Risks

If the sanding is carried out too deeply into the dermis, scarring can result, just as it can with deep chemical peels. Hypopigmentation—the loss of normal pigment color—or hyperpigmentation—dark spots and patches—can also occur.

As with deeper chemical peels and laser resurfacing procedures, it is imperative that patients have been off Accutane for at least six and preferably eighteen months before undergoing dermabrasion. Accutane, an antiacne medication, causes atrophy of the structures embedded in the skin. Because new skin grows from these structures after outer layers of skin are removed, significant scarring can occur after any of these procedures if these structures are missing because of Accutane therapy.

Technique

Dermabrasion is a very operator-sensitive technique. The depth of sanding is determined by the pressure at which the operator holds the burr against the face and by the amount of time the skin is exposed to the abrasive burr. The abrasion continues into the dermis, correcting wrinkles and scars. A full-face dermabrasion will usually take about an hour.

If performed on a small area, local anesthesia suffices. If larger areas are treated, the patient may require intravenous sedation, as well as local anesthesia. Some surgeons however, prefer general anesthesia.

Recovery

The skin that has just undergone dermabrasion should be treated with cleanser and antibiotic ointment. Failure to use ointments will result in drying and crusting, which can be quite tight and uncomfortable. Prescribed medication can control the burning skin pain.

The skin is red and crusted for several days after dermabrasion. The area heals by forming a new outer layer of skin, usually within seven to ten days. The new skin is quite pink and tender. This pinkness will fade over a three-month period, by which time the skin should return to its normal color. The skin texture should be significantly smoother.

Individuals may be more prone to developing inclusion cysts or whiteheads, which can be removed with an abrasive pad or removed with a needle by the surgeon. If patients develop scars, the scars should be aggressively treated with silicone elastomer—which acts as organic, rubberlike material—and steroids for topical use or for injection into scars.

Once the skin is healed after fourteen days, it can be covered with cosmetics. The patient's skin will be more sensitive and prone to irritation from topical agents than before. The patients must avoid sun exposure in the initial weeks after treatment and should use sunblock effective against UVA and UVB with an SPF of thirty or greater on a long-term basis.

Resurfacing Laser

Laser resurfacing has two benefits: It removes the outer layers of skin, penetrating the dermis as with deep chemical peels and dermabrasion. It also shrinks the collagen fibers, thereby tightening the skin.

As skin heals from laser treatment, it is more organized and rejuvenated. New cells form and create a smoother, tighter, and more youthful-appearing skin surface than existed before. Blemishes and pigmented spots are faded, and wrinkles should be significantly improved. The fine wrinkles next to the eyes and wrinkles above the root of the nose respond best to laser resurfacing. The wrinkles in the cheek area respond well. The wrinkles around the lips and mouth are the most difficult to correct; however, there should be a significant improvement even in this area. Acne scars can be significantly improved with the laser technique, although deeply depressed scars cannot be corrected entirely. As with all resurfacing procedures, patients must not have taken Accutane for at least six and preferably eighteen months. Patients with deep wrinkles and depressed scars such as those seen in acne may be best treated in two or more stages.

A nonfractionated laser treatment is a significant medical procedure that should be undertaken only by highly qualified physicians who have been trained in the use of resurfacing lasers. Because the laser resurfacing procedure is carried out in an operating environment by a highly qualified individual, it is relatively expensive, ranging from $1,200 to $2,500 for resurfacing of part of the face and $3,000 to $5,000 for the entire face. The risks, recovery, discomfort, and cost can be reduced by fractionating the laser, as discussed below, but a series of treatments is recommended when converting to fractionated laser treatments.

Laser resurfacing is frequently accomplished with the carbon dioxide (CO_2) laser, Nd:YAG laser, or Erbium:YAG laser. The lasers commonly used today are outlined below.

❖ IPL, or intense pulsed light, is not actually laser light. In fact, it is a broad, unfocused group of wavelengths, often referred to as BBL, or broad band light. It can be used to treat many dermatological conditions, including areas of hyperpigmentation, small blood vessels, excessive oil production, and very fine wrinkles, but its use for resurfacing the face is limited.

❖ Erbium:YAG targets water and is sublative; that is, it only ablates the epidermis rather than into the dermis, much as a superficial chemical peel does, but it also targets and ablates collagen, augmenting the rejuvenation of the skin. This coherent (focused) light targets water with a 2940 nm wavelength laser and collagen with the 3030 nm wavelength.

❖ Neodymium-doped YAG (Nd:YAG) targets melanin in the dermis and ablates the dermis and epidermis. It also effectively treats blood vessels. It is a coherent laser light with a wavelength of 1064 nm.

❖ The carbon dioxide (CO_2) laser targets water and ablates the skin surfaces one at a time. The first pass largely ablates the epidermis. With cleansing between passes, each pass treats a deeper layer of the skin. However, because of the loss of water in the skin with each pass, the laser can damage tissues that were not targeted, so increased risks of hypopigmentation and scarring are possible. CO_2 is a coherent laser light of 10,400 nm wavelength.

❖ In a pulsed mode, a short pulse of light is delivered to the skin at intervals of tiny fractions of a second. Less heat transfers to the tissue, so the effect can be limited to the superficial layers of the skin. The energy can be adjusted: The longer the pulse, the deeper the penetration is. This is beneficial in that longer pulses can be used for thicker skin; moreover, the physician can discern and control the desired depth of penetration.

Fractionated Lasers

Fractionated lasers are now increasing in popularity. These lasers do not ablate all areas of the skin that are treated with a laser. Instead, they pass through the epidermis to target particular areas in the dermis. These less traumatic techniques minimize procedural pain and downtime. Redness, the healing process, and peeling are usually negligible. However, the overall benefit is less and multiple treatments are required, typically five to ten laser treatments at monthly intervals.

Technique

The skin may be pretreated for two weeks with tretinoin or alpha hydroxy acids. The patient is also usually pretreated with antiviral medications to prevent eruption of cold sores (herpes simplex) in the resurfaced skin.

The patient is placed lying faceup and given sedation either orally or intravenously. Anesthesia can be applied to the skin topically or by blocking the major facial nerves with Xylocaine. Some surgeons use conscious sedation or general anesthesia. Eye protection is then applied. The laser probe is passed back and forth over the skin as the laser light vaporizes the top layers of skin. There may be areas of residual sensation, and it feels as though one is being hit with a snapping rubber band. When the laser is applied to the skin, the patient may smell smoke as it is being removed by a smoke evacuator.

Before a second pass is completed, the vaporized skin can be removed in areas where there is thicker skin or a greater need. This procedure can be repeated until a level is reached at which the wrinkles are corrected. Depending on the type of laser to be used and the area to be resurfaced, the procedure can last over an hour. The deeper the resurfacing, the longer the recovery time will be.

Recovery

At the end of the procedure, the skin is red, raw, and crusted. The vaporized skin can be left in place as a biological dressing. The face may be dressed with an occlusive dressing, or a topical gel. There are no steadfast rules as to how to keep the face dressed. Some surgeons will remove dressings after forty-eight hours and continue with topical gels. Others prefer to change the dressing every two days for a seven to ten days, while still others will leave the dressing in place for a week or so, until it separates. Proponents of prolonged dressings believe that it keeps the skin moist and more comfortable. Some patients are unable to wear dressings because of associated claustrophobia.

The face will generally heal within ten to fourteen days. The skin will remain a pink red to a bright red for a minimum of several weeks. In most patients, this redness persists for two to four months. It is imperative to avoid sun exposure during this period. Sunblocks must be applied whenever the patient is out in sunlight. Failure to follow these guidelines can result in areas of hyperpigmentation that manifest as dark spots and blotches. Darker complexions carry greater risk of developing hyperpigmentation. Should this occur, patients may be treated immediately with alternating applications of tretinoin (a vitamin A-derived exfoliant) and hydroquinone (a bleaching agent).

Patients may develop scarring in areas that are subjected to too deep a laser. These areas must be aggressively treated with silicone elastomer, a piece of silicone that is placed on the scar. Although the mechanism is poorly understood, the constant pressure from the silicone helps scars flatten and blend with surrounding tissues. If silicone by itself is not adequate to treat scars, cortisone injections into the scarred areas, given one month apart for three to four months, can greatly improve the final outcome.

In the initial months after laser treatment, the skin is usually dryer and more sensitive to topical agents than it was before. Some patients find that moisturizers that were well tolerated previously now cause irritation. This problem should resolve within several months.

The Face: Recontouring the Soft Tissues

Botulinum Toxin (i.e., Botox Cosmetic, Dysport, Xeomin)

Botulinum toxin is known best as the first commercially available Botox (*OnabotulinumtoxinA*), but there are several commonly used types. Xeomin (*IncobotulinumtoxinA*) is used very similarly but is felt to diffuse a bit more. Dysport (*AbobotulinumtoxinA*) works similarly but requires approximately three times as many units as Botox and Xeomin so the cost per unit is significantly less. Botulinum toxin is released by the bacterium *Clostridium botulinum* and prevents nerves from stimulating muscles to contract, so muscles are weak or flaccid. Hyperactive muscles are frequently treated with botulinum toxin as their contraction create certain, typical furrows. (See Figure 13.)

Botulinum toxin has been used since the 1990s to relieve abnormal muscle spasms. However, it was soon discovered that it helped with wrinkles and signs of photoaging. It is not FDA-approved for many of the uses for which it is being used off-label. Eight distinct toxins have been found, but only botulinum toxin A is FDA-approved for treating abnormal facial muscle spasms; eyelid and eye muscle problems called blepharospasm and strabismus; and axillary hyperhydrosis, or excessive sweating under the armpits.

So that the effect is localized, minute amounts of toxin are injected only into the intended muscle. Injected botulinum toxin weakens the overactive muscle contractions, causing a flattening in the area and improved appearance. The injected muscle cannot pull the overlying skin into a wrinkle. Competing muscles also do not have to work as hard, leading to additional smoothing in some areas not treated. This effect is very different from the illness seen in patients afflicted with systemic botulism poisoning: Botulism patients have massive amounts of toxin circulating throughout the bloodstream, causing a loss of muscle function all over the body. This is a potentially fatal illness. In contrast, no long-term adverse effects or health hazards from controlled injections of botulinum toxin have been described to date. Patients who have had long-term treatment with botulinum toxin may develop antibodies, which do not cause any problems but can make all future injections ineffective. Sequential treatments are necessary to maintain the antiwrinkle effect.

Most individuals have been very happy with the injections. Beneficial effects are seen within one to three days and can last four to six months. Efficacy is reported to be in the 95% range, and 64% of individuals report satisfactory results for three months or longer. Costs are usually done by unit ($9 to $18 per unit for Botox and Xeomin or $3 to $6 per unit for Dysport) or by treatment area ($200 to $400 per area).

Technique

Botox and Xeomin come in 100-unit vials of purified botulinum A toxin. Dysport comes in 300-unit vials. It is mixed with 0.5 mg of human albumin and 0.9 mg of sodium chloride (salt water). At the physician's office, it is reconstituted with 1 mL to 5 mL of sterile water to give a variable concentration of botulinum for each 0.1 mL of solution. There is some variability between different physician techniques.

The needle is placed through the skin over the wrinkle or exaggerated crease, and the toxin injected in small aliquots (equal portions of the vial that leave no remainder). Botulinum toxin is most commonly used at the forehead, the glabellar area (junction between the forehead and nose), the nasolabial crease (junction between the upper lip and the cheek), the "bunny lines" (areas at the sides of the nose), the crow's feet (areas adjacent to the eyes), the dimpled chin, and the neck bands (see figure 13). Physicians may massage treatment areas, but the patient should not.

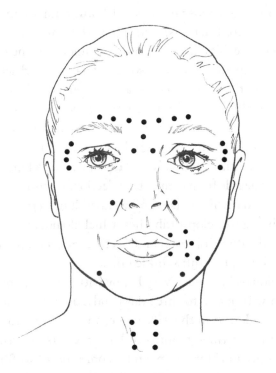

Figure 13. Botulinum toxin frequent injection sites in the face

Exercising the muscles for a few hours after the injections are complete may expedite the toxin's effects. Side effects may occur at the injection site and include pain and bruising, which are usually very short-lived and can be limited by applying ice after the injection. Occasionally, patients have reported headache after injection, but this is exceedingly rare. In actuality, more patients see improvement in their headaches than the opposite scenario due to muscle relaxation. Sometimes the toxin can diffuse to adjacent muscles, causing unwanted weakness in these muscles. These side effects can be most noticeable around the eye: Any weakness of the upper-eyelid muscles leads to upper-eyelid drooping. Just as the desired effects are temporary, these adverse side effects are as well.

Fat Injection

In the face, fat injections are used to treat deep wrinkles, depressions, skin folds, and areas of fat atrophy. This technique has also become quite popular for lip-plumping procedures. In other areas of the body, fat can be used (1) to augment the breast or buttock, (2) to correct deficiencies of the body contour that grew during childhood and adolescent development or were caused by other surgeries, or (3) to thicken areas that have become deficient with age (especially the back of the hand or the areas around the eyes).

Fat injection is advantageous because there are no risks of an allergic reaction or rejection of foreign material—the fat came from the patient's own body. Moreover, the injected fat tends to be longer-lasting than foreign material. The technique does not necessarily provide a permanent solution, as the body reabsorbs some fat over the first year (30%–70% in different reports); this reabsorption may lead to irregularities in appearance. Some fat stem cells are transplanted to help grow new fat cells; these can remain viable permanently.

Unwanted effects may include redness at the injection site for several days and an uneven distribution of fat after the procedure. Because fat injection also involves fat harvest and preparation, it is fairly expensive, ranging between $700 and $4,000, depending on the number and size of the areas being treated.

Technique

Fat is taken directly from a donor site on the body or removed with a liposuction device, generally from the buttock, thighs, or lower abdomen. The fat is then prepared in one of a variety of ways. Many surgeons filter the fat through a cheesecloth. Others centrifuge the fat to remove blood cells and serum. In addition, many commercial products are now available to help capture, cleanse, and prepare the fat for injection. Some evidence suggests that the fat is longer-lasting if it is mixed with the patient's blood serum. To accomplish this, a sample of blood can be taken from a vein and prepared in a centrifuge. The serum can be removed from the red blood cells and mixed with the fat. As the new mixture of fat and serum spins in the centrifuge, the lighter fat comes to the surface. It is carefully removed from the serum below the surface and placed in a syringe for injection. The physician must be careful to avoid injecting fat into a blood vessel.

Resorbable Fillers

These fillers are deemed resorbable because the body will reabsorb them over time, and, in general, are shorter-lasting than fat as a filler. The resorbable, injectable fillers available are bovine collagen, human-derived skin fillers, and other synthetic or natural materials.

TYPE	DURATION	SKIN TEST
Bovine Collagen		
Zyderm®	3 - 6 months	X
Zyderm II®		
Zyplast®		
Human Collagen		
CosmoDerm I™		
CosmoDerm II™	3 - 6 months	
CosmoPlast™		
Porcine Collagen		
Evolence®	6 months	
Hyaluronic Acid		
Restylane®	6 months	
Perlane™	6 - 9 months	
Juvederm Ultra®	6 -12 months	
Juvederm Ultra Plus®	9 -12 months	
Hylaform®	3 - 6 months	
Captique™	4 months	
Puragen™	6 months	
Polymethyl methacrylate with Bovine Collagen		
Artefill®	Permanent	X
Poly-L-Lactic Acid		
Sculptra®	12 months	
Calcium Hydroxylapatite		
Radiesse®	12 months	

Figure 14. Resorbable fillers with their components, duration, and allergy-testing needs

The most problematic complication that can occur with injection of fat or any of the fillers below is injection into a blood vessel, which can lead to an embolism. A peripheral embolism can cause death of local tissues or blindness if it occurs near the eyes, although this is exceedingly rare.

Bovine Collagen

Collagen, for many years, was the main option for soft-tissue augmentation. The first collagen products were made from purified, sterile, bovine collagen harvested from cow skin. Zyderm I is 3.5% bovine collagen and is used for superficial wrinkles. Zyderm II has a higher concentration (6.5%) of collagen, is therefore thicker, and is used for medium wrinkles. Zyplast is cross-linked with glutaraldehyde, which makes it more resistant to breakdown and less likely to trigger an immune response. Zyplast is better than Zyderm for deep wrinkles and folds and for lip augmentation. All the products are premixed with dilute, local anesthetic (lidocaine).

Both Zyderm and Zyplast are slowly reabsorbed; correction of wrinkles typically lasts for a maximum of three to four months, and oftentimes the correction lasts only six to eight weeks. As the collagen reabsorbs, the wrinkle reappears, and reinjection is needed. One cubic centimeter of collagen, at a cost of about $400, will treat multiple fine wrinkles.

Risks

Three percent of the population is highly allergic to either the cow-derived collagen protein or the additives in the solution. Thus, it is imperative that every patient undergo an allergy test before treatment. A small dose of Zyderm or Zyplast (0.1 mL) is injected into the forearm, and if, after four weeks, there is any redness or swelling, the individual is considered allergic and is not a candidate for use of these products in the future. It is advisable and safer to give two test doses three weeks apart; the final determination then is delayed until four weeks after injection of the second dose. Doctors recommend retesting if more than a year has elapsed since the last treatment.

Technique

The collagen is injected into the wrinkle or crease. The injection is placed into the dermis because material injected more deeply, into the subcutaneous tissue, is reabsorbed rapidly. When injecting Zyderm, the wrinkle must be overcorrected, as the water in Zyderm will be absorbed by the body. The procedure is typically not painful because lidocaine is part of the product, although a topical anesthetic may be applied.

Recovery and Side Effects

After injection of Zyderm, the area is red and swollen for several hours. Zyplast does not contain water, and so the area tends not to be swollen following injection. If the injection is excessive in one area, the skin may be too high. If the injection is too deep, there will be rapid absorption and disappearance of the collagen. Bacterial infection or bruising may occur. There are few side effects for a patient who is not allergic to bovine collagen.

Human-Derived Skin Fillers

Several skin fillers can be made from human tissues: collagen protein, dermis, and fascia. These fillers do not contain any cells, so immune rejection of foreign tissue does not occur. The products are tested for known diseases caused by viruses and bacteria.

The major advantage of dermal fillers is the decreased number of allergic reactions they cause. In contrast to bovine collagen, human collagen should not cause an allergic reaction; however, some have been reported and are due most likely to a preservative in the product. As a result, skin testing is not recommended by the manufacturer but may be performed by some physicians.

Dermalogen is a collagen matrix filler derived from the skin of cadavers. It is tested for the viral diseases HIV and hepatitis and then treated to prevent disease transmission from bacteria, viruses, and prions (foreign proteins that act as infectious agents). The product may last slightly longer (three to four months) than bovine collagen, but sequential injections are recommended (typically three injections given over several weeks). The increased costs over bovine collagen (between $500 and $800 per cc) limit its use at present.

Autologen is manufactured in the same way as Dermalogen, but it is prepared from a patient's own skin. It requires an initial procedure to harvest skin and then several weeks of processing time. The costs can be significant ($2,000 to $4,000 per batch), but the skin can be stored and used for the series of three to four treatments that are typically necessary. Despite being from a patient's own body, the injected collagen is ultimately degraded by the body, like other collagen injections. The filler lasts three to six months.

CosmoDerm and CosmoPlast are collagen matrices harvested from circumcised neonatal foreskin. CosmoPlast is more resistant to breakdown and has greater cross-linking than CosmoDerm, making it better for deeper wrinkles. Cost is about $400 to $800 per cc, and usually a dose of 1 cc–2 cc is used. The effects last three to six months.

Cymetra consists of small particles of AlloDerm, which is a proprietary preparation of human dermis. This product contains the matrix and the collagen of the dermis, encouraging beneficial ingrowth of the patient's nearby tissue. However, the effects of Cymetra are still temporary, lasting three to six months.

Fascian is a particulate product that is harvested and manufactured from the fascia tissue around muscles from the extremities of cadavers. It can be injected to correct wrinkles and grooves, but unfortunately, it is thick and difficult to inject. Its effects also last three to six months.

Other Injectable Fillers, Synthetic or Natural

Hyaluronic Acid

The use of hyaluronic acid as a dermal filler has become a huge component of cosmetic surgery and dermatology care. Hyaluronic acid products are frequently used for fine wrinkles, lips, smile lines, and creases around the mouth by injecting in the mid-dermis. Hyaluronic acid is a glycosaminoglycan, which is a normal component of skin and other parts of the human body; it is important in skin hydration. Its presence attracts water, which thickens skin in the area of injection.

The major advantages of hyaluronic acid over fat and the human-derived dermal products are (1) the ability to make a thin liquid that is much easier to inject, especially in superficial, fine wrinkles and (2) its ready-to-use preparation. Because it is a naturally occurring substance, an allergic reaction to hyaluronic acid is not possible. It is, however, possible to have an allergic reaction to a preservative in a particular product.

The variety of products available has different sources, preparations, and durability. The products' effectiveness typically lasts from six to twelve months (see table). Trade names include Restylane, Perlane, Juvéderm, Xeomin, Hylaform, Reviderm Intra, AcHyal, and Belotero. Some details are given below:

- Hylaform is produced from the combs of roosters, so a person with allergies to other bird proteins or eggs may also be allergic to Hylaform. Its effects last approximately nine months.
- Restylane and Juvéderm are stable, partially cross-linked hyaluronic acid derived from bacteria called streptococcus (not an animal source), so they do not possess the allergic risk that bird-derived fillers have. Its effects last six to nine months.
- Perlane is a larger molecule of hyaluronic acid that is used for deeper augmentation and whose effects last longer than the other products' do (nine to twelve months).
- Reviderm Intra is another bacterial hyaluronic acid that is combined with dextran beads, which are felt to promote collagen production. It is effective for superficial wrinkles but is currently unavailable in the United States.
- Voluma is a newer HA that is thicker and lasts longer, up to two years, but it must be injected deeper and is less forgiving of a filler.
- Belotero is a newer, thinner HA that can be used in finer wrinkles and thinner skin.

Typical costs range from $400 to $1000 per treatment. Topical anesthetic or nerve field blocks are frequently used, unless the product is premixed with lidocaine. Most complications are related to pain, irritation, or bruising, which should resolve within days. As with all fillers, more significant risks are related to poor injection technique, which either causes the result to look less beautiful or, more seriously, leads to scarring. Therefore, a patient should be treated by a properly trained professional, such as a plastic surgeon, even though the technique is minimally invasive.

Lactic Acid

Sculptra (known in Europe as New-Fill) is FDA-approved for restoring the loss of facial fat in patients with AIDS (acquired immunodeficiency syndrome). It consists of a synthetic form of lactic acid that is biocompatible, does not trigger an immune response, and recruits beneficial collagen ingrowth.

The effects are not immediate but cumulative. Typically, three or four treatments are needed about every three to four months to gradually increase the thickness of the skin and the face. After a series of treatments, the effect has provided significant improvement in facial appearance for over two years. The cost of $600 to $1,000 per session can be prohibitive.

Calcium Hydroxyapatite

Radiesse/Radiance FN is a long-lasting (two- to three-year) injectable filler made with calcium hydroxyapatite, a material found in normal bone. It stimulates new collagen growth. This filler does not require skin testing because it is biocompatible (which means that it is compatible with human tissues and does not cause any injury or immune response). Unfortunately, there have been reports of inconsistency of filler material and significant inflammatory reactions, which have limited its use by some plastic surgeons. The cost is also significant, at $800 to $2,500.

Permanent Fillers

Silicone

Silicone has many manufacturers. This synthetic polymer will not react with the body; it comes in many different forms and viscosities. Solid forms, in contrast to porous forms, do not allow ingrowth of the patient's own tissue, making it more likely that the material will migrate, leak, exit the skin (in a complication called extrusion), or become infected. Over the years, using silicone has frequently been complicated by inconsistencies. Other problems occur when the body surrounds the silicone with abnormal growths of white blood cells attempting to contain the silicone, called granulomas. Sometimes, patients have needed surgical removal of the material.

Silicone's use as a cosmetic filler was outlawed by the FDA. Still, many people use it off-label for cosmetic purposes (Silikon 1000). The cost ranges from $100 to $1,000, depending on the material's formulation.

Gore-Tex, or Polytetrafluoroethylene (PTFE)

Gore-Tex, or polytetrafluoroethylene (PTFE), is available in a tube and is known as SoftForm). This injectable material features more ingrowth of the patient's own skin tissue than silicone does. It is permanent but, unfortunately, prone to extrusion from the skin, as well as to infection, granulomas (white blood cell growths, as described above), migration, and palpability (the ability to feel the injected material below the skin). The cost of the injection ranges from $500 to $1,500.

Collagen and Polymethylmethacrylate Combinations

Combinations of bovine collagen and polymethylmethacrylate are sold as Artecoll and Arteplast. These products are used for deeper wrinkles, grooves, and soft-tissue deficiencies. Polymethylmethacrylate is frequently used for skull remodeling; it is the permanent component of the product because it is too large for the immune system to remove. The filler works well in two ways: (1) immediately, because its larger particles create bulk, and (2) permanently, because it recruits new collagen deposits from the patient's own skin. Overcorrection is not necessary with these products.

While the permanence of Artecoll and Arteplast is an advantage, it is also a problem if inconsistencies exist, if superficial (shallow) injection leads to beading or if granulomas form. The deeper these products are injected, the less likely these complications are to be visible above the skin. The bovine collagen ingredient means that patients require skin testing before use. The cost is approximately $600 to $800 per syringe, and one to three syringes are typically used in a session. In addition to these permanent fillers, different products may be needed to fill more superficial wrinkles.

Implants

Implants are used in a multitude of applications to bolster skin where tissue is lacking. The insertion of implants requires a true surgical procedure to place the implant. It also carries more risk than injection procedures do.

Surgical exposure of the location where the implant is to be placed may cause bleeding and injury to the body's anatomy. In addition, a foreign object in the body is at risk for infection, misplaced position, extrusion, and migration. The type of implanted material determines the relative risk of such procedures.

Silicone

Silicone, as mentioned in the filler section, has been around for many years. It was originally developed by Dow Corning Corporation and has many different formulations and costs (ranging from less than $100 to more than $2,000). It can be ordered in standard or custom-molded shapes that fill in defects shown on a template or radiographic image. Its use is limited by the typical complications of palpability, granulomas, infection, extrusion, and migration.

Gore-Tex, or Polytetrafluoroethylene (PTFE)

Gore-Tex, also known as polytetrafluoroethylene (PTFE), comes in various forms that are ready to implant: sutures, sheets, forms, and patches. As mentioned before, Gore-Tex is inert but prone to the same typical complications of extrusion, infection, palpability, granulomas, and migration. The cost of the implant ranges from $500 to $2,000, in addition to the cost of the surgical procedure.

Medpor

Medpor (Porex Surgical Inc., College Park, Georgia) is a porous, high-density polyethylene implant that comes premolded or custom-made. The advantage of Medpor over Gore-Tex and silicone is its porous structure, which allows ingrowth of structural tissue that contains blood vessels. This ingrowth stabilizes the implant—which limits migration and extrusion—and decrease of infection. The cost of the implants is variable, but is typically $500 to $2,500, in addition to the surgical fee.

Acellular Dermal Matrices

Acellular dermal matrices, such as Cymetra created from AlloDerm discussed in the fillers section above, can also be used as a graft or implant. It is created from the dermis of cadavers by a (remove proprietary) process that removes all skin cells and treats all known potential sources of disease and infection. Sheets of ADM can be used to augment features, correct soft tissue deficits, or reconstruct structural anatomy. ADM is often used in lip augmentation, where it is inserted rolled up under lip mucosa. It is also frequently used to fill in areas of atrophy or depression and to correct surgical-scar depressions. ADM acts as a matrix: it is ultimately supplied with blood vessels and is infiltrated and incorporated by nearby cells. Infection, migration, and extrusion are not a significant problem with ADM, as they are with permanent implants.

Conclusions

There is a variety of minimally invasive techniques to rejuvenate the skin and other soft tissues. Skin resurfacing removes the epidermis and varying layers of the dermis to relieve the aging effects of time, environmental, and sun damage. Superficial signs of aging include fine wrinkles, altered pigmentation, skin laxity, clogged pores, and hyperkeratosis (thickened skin). Skin resurfacing can be accomplished with chemical peels, dermabrasion, or laser resurfacing, all of which can be done to any skin depth.

With time, the soft tissues of the face atrophy and fall because of the effects of gravity, creating deep wrinkles in the face and loss of the youthful shape of the face. Significant soft-tissue changes require standard surgical techniques, but many minimally invasive techniques exist, and many more are being developed. Botox is used to relax muscles that contribute to wrinkles and downward change. Fillers are used to correct fine to medium wrinkles. Most available products last a mere three to nine months, whereas most permanent or semipermanent fillers harbor significant risks. The perfect filler would be permanent, stay in place, and cause no immune response; however, such a material has not yet been developed. Filler materials and Botox are often combined for the variety of rejuvenation needs in a face. Fat injection is used for larger, deeper wrinkles and areas of depression or tissue deficit. Implants are used for more significant deficits but also require more invasive procedures.

FACE-LIFTS: SURGICAL
REJUVENATION OF THE AGING FACE

The continuous and relentless aging process typically becomes apparent in the face around forty years of age and is very evident as one ages into the fifties and sixties. Age-related changes do not simply reflect changes in the skin itself: Aging also causes an overall loss of bulk in the skin. The skin becomes thinner than it was before, its texture becomes coarse, and the subcutaneous fat slowly disappears. As the skin, fat, muscle, and attachments to bone weaken and stretch, gravity causes these soft tissues to sag. Meanwhile, the bones of the face and skull stay in the same place, so the skin loses its youthful fit on the face. Muscles also create furrows as they repeatedly pull the skin over many decades.

Genetic factors largely determine the age at which fine wrinkles, deep creases, and furrows become apparent and the rate at which they grow, but lifestyle and environmental exposure also play important roles. Cigarette smoking and the ultraviolet radiation from chronic sun exposure, both of which are cumulative over one's lifetime, lead to the most dramatic changes in skin. Factors such as stress, alcoholism, chronic illness, and certain medications also encourage the aging process.

Facial rejuvenation procedures, both surgical and nonsurgical, address all these processes. They can turn back the clock, but they will not stop the aging process. After treatment, the clock starts ticking again, and the signs of aging continue to develop.

Candidates for a Face-Lift

No age requirements exist for face-lift operations. Clearly, a young person who lacks the classic features of aging should wait until a correctable, defined problem exists, but early treatment can limit the severity of age-related changes in appearance and improve the overall outcome. The benefits of early, preventive treatment have become even more evident with the increasingly popular, less invasive options. Preventive treatments are best for patients under forty who understand that these techniques do not eliminate the need for later surgical rejuvenation as changes occur in the deeper tissue layers of the face.

A healthy person has no upper-age limit for facial cosmetic surgery; rejuvenation procedures can be safely performed on patients in their eighties. The majority of facial rejuvenation operations are performed in individuals in their forties, fifties, and sixties.

Some face-lift procedures have earned popular and marketing-oriented names, such as "lunchtime lifts," "short-scar face-lifts," and "weekend face-lifts." Descriptions of these are at the end of this chapter under the section entitled "Alternative Face-Lift Procedures." So that the reader can understand how a face-lift moves the different structures of the face, an explanation of the typical signs of aging and the traditional face-lift procedures is given first.

Specific Causes of the Signs of Facial Aging

Sagging Skin and Wrinkling

The drawings below show the results of common aging processes that occur in the face: sagging skin and soft tissue combined with deep wrinkles caused by muscle activity.

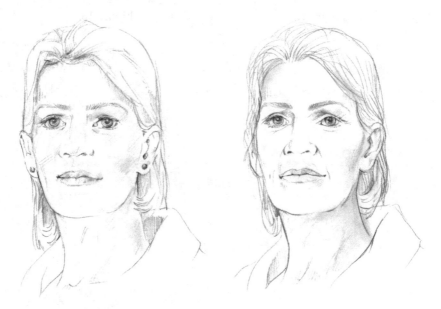

Figure 15   Figure 16

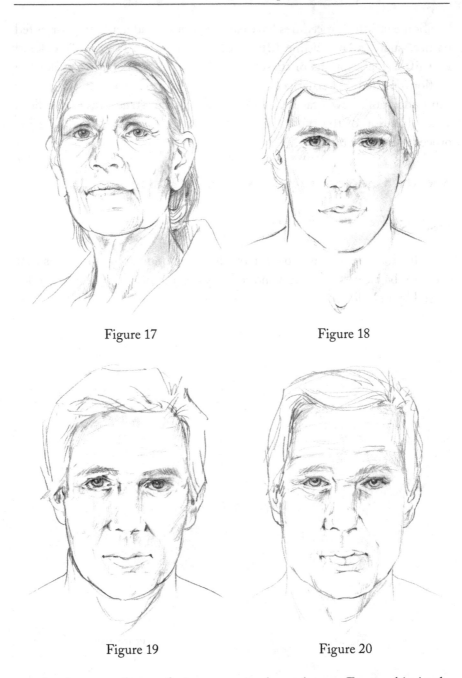

Figure 17

Figure 18

Figure 19

Figure 20

In the upper face, soft tissue sags in the eyebrows. Excess skin in the upper and lower eyelids loses its elasticity and definition, causing it to hang. Weakening of the deeper tissues in the eyelids allow the fat behind the eyelids to pouch outward. Then, muscles of the face work deep wrinkles and creases into the skin and deeper soft tissue. Hyperactive muscles that oppose gravitational pull create certain typical furrows. (See table.)

Location	Description	Wrinkle Direction	Muscle Name
Forehead	Above eyebrows	Horizontal	Frontalis
Upper glabella	Between eyebrows, above nose	Vertical	Corrugator
Lower glabella	Just above nose	Horizontal	Procerus
Crow's-feet area	Between lower eyelid and temple	Horizontal	Orbicularis oculi

Deep wrinkles of the upper face and the muscles that cause them

Aging in the cheeks and jowls also shows both sagging and wrinkling. Skin and fat over the cheekbone (the malar area or midface) begin to sag, creating heaviness and depth in a deep wrinkle between the upper lip and cheek (the nasolabial fold). The jowls become heavy at the corner of the jawbone, as one ligament weakens and another takes over: The masseteric cutaneous retaining ligament weakens, so the mandibular facial retaining ligament, a strong soft-tissue connection to bone, holds up the descending instead.

The fat below the face and, specifically, below the chin becomes more prominent with aging, and excess skin begins to hang from the neck. Vertical bands form down the neck because the superficial (shallow) muscle of the neck, called the platysma, begins to tighten. There are also gravitational effects on the nose, ears, lips, and chin.

Genetic, Environmental, and Weight Factors

Some individuals carry genes that cause an early appearance of an aged face or even of a single feature, changes that are not necessarily attributable to aging. It is common to see younger individuals or a group of relatives with extremely lax lower eyelids and a protrusion of fat behind the lid that causes bags or festoons due to a hereditary laxity of the orbital septum. Other individuals may have excess neck skin and fat that create the classic "turkey gobbler deformity" even at an early or thin stage.

Patients with massive weight loss—such as that frequently seen after gastric bypass surgery—endure exaggerated changes. Obesity stretches the ligaments, muscles, and skin, which have a difficult time returning to a youthful position as the fat goes away.

The Traditional Face-Lift

A face-lift, known as a rhytidectomy, is designed to tighten the skin of the lower face and neck by removing excess skin and newly suspending the face from the support structures underneath it. A face-lift tightens the loosely hanging skin in the neck and jowls, corrects the frown-like downturn of skin at the corner of the mouth, and reduces the depth of the nasolabial fold by reversing the descent of cheek skin toward the mouth if the midface is addressed. A surgeon can perform a "midface lift" simultaneously or separately from a traditional, lower face-lift, which does not alter the cheeks. Although a face-lift does not correct fine wrinkles on the skin, general facial improvement can be dramatic. Facial resurfacing can address the superficial wrinkles in deteriorated skin by removing damaged layers of skin to replace them with tighter, more youthful skin (see chapter on minimally invasive facial procedures).

The most common facial rejuvenation procedures and the other enhancements often combined with face-lifts include the following:

- Face-lift of the lower face (rhytidectomy)
- Midface lift of the cheek area
- Cheek augmentation of firm cheek structures
- Neck lift of soft neck tissues
- Forehead and brow lift
- Eyelid surgery (blepharoplasty), upper or lower
- Nasal reconstruction surgery (rhinoplasty)
- Ear surgery (otoplasty)
- Lip surgery (augmentation, lifts, and reductions)
- Chin surgery (implants and reshaping through genioplasty)
- Minimally invasive procedures (Botox, fillers, and skin resurfacing)

Surgeons may perform individual procedures or a combination of techniques for an overall facial rejuvenation.

Consultation

Before consultation, patients should have a general understanding of the features and age-related changes that are troublesome to them and the surgical improvements that they would like to achieve. They need to consider how much they are prepared to go through, both surgically and financially. By combining this understanding with the knowledge and expertise of a board-certified plastic surgeon, an appropriate plan can be formulated between the patient and surgeon.

In the consultations before surgery, the surgeon carefully obtains a thorough medical history. If a patient has a chronic illness such as heart disease, high blood pressure, or diabetes, the surgeon may require the patient to have a preoperative consultation with a family physician or internist to ensure that elective surgery is safe.

Medications that interfere with clotting (for example, over the counter aspirin and NSAIDs or prescription anticoagulants such as Coumadin and Plavix) can lead to excessive bleeding, so they must be stopped ten days before the operation. The degree of bruising and the amount of time it takes for it to disappear is also quite variable, so any history of easy bruising should be discussed.

A patient should thoroughly and honestly report tobacco use. This honesty is critical because cigarette smokers have a reduced blood supply to their skin that causes a higher incidence of incision-healing complications. In fact, some surgeons will not operate on cigarette smokers at all. Most surgeons will still operate on smokers but require several weeks or months of nicotine avoidance both before and after surgery.

There are many variations on face-lift techniques, but in most surgeons' hands, the procedure lasts between two and four hours. It may be carried out as an outpatient operation in the surgeon's office or operating facility, an outpatient surgical facility, or a hospital operating room. Some surgeons use intravenous sedation with local anesthesia, and some surgeons prefer a general anesthetic, where the patient is asleep.

Technique

For surgery, the patient is laid on his or her back on the operating table. The patient's head will be slightly raised and the face or the scalp fully cleansed to allow the surgeon to turn the face and make side-to-side comparisons. If the patient is not heavily sedated or asleep, anesthetizing the face with needle injections may cause discomfort. Patients who have been sedated normally experience very little pain and rarely remember this portion of the procedure. Once the face is numb, the sedation level may be reduced to increase the patient's safety. At this point, the patient may feel head-turning, pressure, or occasional pulling but should feel no pain or discomfort.

There are many named but similar techniques, so each surgeon has a unique regimen for the operation. Even the typical incisions display only minor variability (see figure 21).

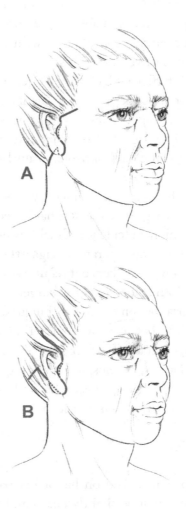

Figure 21. Illustrations of typical face-lift incisions

The surgeon performs the upper incision either at the hairline or in the hair-bearing temple above the ear. From there, it travels downward, just in front of the top half of the ear. Some surgeons prefer to hide the scar by carrying the incision slightly into the ear behind the tragus (the flat projection of cartilage in front of the ear that can be pressed to block sound). Other surgeons leave the incision in front of the tragus to prevent blunting its appearance. To avoid bringing bearded skin into the ear, the surgeon usually places the incision in front of the tragus in men. The incision then extends below the earlobe and along or near the crease behind the ear, where it joins the skull. From behind the ear, it may travel into the hair-bearing scalp in one of a variety of patterns. Rejuvenating the neck without leaving scars requires careful, skillful technique in this extremely visible area.

Most commonly, the surgeon will use several tools to lift the skin of the face and neck off the subcutaneous fat and muscles that lie just underneath it. Once the skin has been lifted, a layer of muscles and fibrous material known as the SMAS is identified. The SMAS connects the superficial platysma muscle of the neck with the fascia layer of the scalp that lies deep below the soft tissue at the edge of the face. Many surgeons will use permanent sutures to elevate and tighten the SMAS and the back edge of the platysma to provide a firm pull on the deeper structures of the lower face and neck. Lifting these deep structures is the main reason that a face-lift provides a long-lasting youthful appearance to the face and avoids the need to overtighten the skin attempting to support the deep structures. This is key to achieving a natural result. See figure 22.

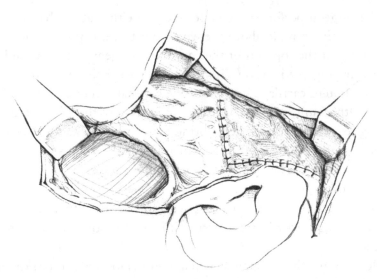

Figure 22: SMAS plication

Once the deep structures are pulled up, the skin must be pulled and fitted to match deeper tissues in a procedural step called redraping. After redraping the elevated skin, the skin is tacked in place with sutures. Then the excess skin is removed. Fixing the redraped skin in its new position above and behind the ears is essential to lifting the face, second in importance only to the deep-layer suspension described immediately above.

The remaining incisions are closed to leave as little tension on the staples or sutures as possible; this technique creates the best, least visible scar. The skin incisions behind and in front of the ear are closed with sutures. The incision in the scalp will be closed with stitches. Early face-lift techniques required skin tension, which led to the "windswept" look that frightens so many patients who desire facial rejuvenation. Today, this look is considered a sign of a poor result.

The surgeon will have controlled any bleeding with sutures or an electrical device that coagulates the small bleeding points. This tool, called a bovie (after its inventor, Dr. William T. Bovie), or bipolar electrocautery device, may make unusual noises or cause the patient to smell smoke during the procedure. The surgeon uses this tool very precisely, so these events should not cause alarm if the patient is awake. A small drainage tube may be placed in the incision around the ear to evacuate any collecting blood or fluid, depending on the amount of bleeding during the procedure or on the surgeon's preference. A drain if placed is typically removed the next day.

Recovery

Typically this is an outpatient operation. However, an overnight stay for observation may be required by some surgeons or for certain patients, depending on preferences, health status, and the surgeon's findings during surgery.

In the initial hours after surgery, the patient may feel facial weakness from the local anesthetic used during surgery. Some anesthetic agents can block nerve communication with muscles of facial expression for several hours. This may lead to weakness in opening and closing the eyes, smiling, puckering the lips, and elevating the brow.

There is surprisingly little pain after surgery of the head and neck. Intravenous (IV) medications and the stress of the surgery may cause a general feeling of illness. Usually, the discomfort of swelling is easily controlled with prescribed medication; it resolves after three to five days.

If drainage tubes were used, they will be removed as soon as fluid drainage stops, usually within one to three days after surgery. The sutures just in front of the ear are removed within a week. The sutures or staples in the temple and behind the ear are usually left in place for three or four days longer because these areas are less visible to others and take longer to heal.

Visible swelling and bruising are inevitable, but sleeping in a semirecumbent or upright position for the first forty-eight hours can reduce this postoperative swelling, as can cool compresses. Most surgeons will place a compression dressing around the face to limit swelling. This dressing will be removed within twenty-four to forty-eight hours. After its removal, gentle showering and washing of hair is safe. The degree of swelling varies among patients and techniques. It can range from mild and barely perceptible to very significant swelling, with the face becoming round and full, often referred to as a "pumpkin." The time each patient needs for the swelling to dissipate also varies. Most of the swelling may resolve within four or five days, but in some individuals, swelling can persist for weeks.

Usually the bruising will resolve adequately by ten to twelve days after surgery. It does descend onto the neck and chest as it resolves.

Activity will be quite limited for the first five to seven days. At ten days, patients begin to feel normal: the stitches will have been removed, and most of the residual bruising can be covered with makeup, and patients should be ready to resume some work and social activity. Most acquaintances and observers probably will not notice anything after $2^1/_2$ to 3 weeks, but close friends and family will see many changes. Strenuous exercise is usually permitted within three to four weeks. The surgeon should guide the patient through an individualized recovery period.

Typical Patient Concerns After Surgery

After the operation and during the initial weeks of the healing process, patients often do not feel that they look good. A patient commonly feels depressed after having gone through discomfort, time, and expense. Most concerns that worry patients are part of the normal healing process. Therefore, it is important for the patient to act patiently and not to be too critical of appearance too soon after surgery. The face-lift operation cannot change basic structure of the bones under the face, nor can it return the appearance of decades before. However, with realistic expectations and good surgical technique, the benefits of a face-lift will soon present themselves. The surgeon and patient should see each other frequently to discuss any concerns that arise.

Many subtle changes continue to take place for several months. The scars will slowly settle, and their red discoloration will fade. Slight asymmetries between the two sides of the face will appear. These occur mainly because faces are not symmetrical even in infancy and further because the swelling and skin relaxation after surgery will be different on each side. There may be scattered areas of firmness as small collections of fluid and blood go through reabsorption and the normal healing process— massage techniques benefit these areas.

Initially, all fine wrinkles will disappear because of the swelling in the skin, but the face-lift operation does not correct fine wrinkles. As the swelling resolves, the fine skin wrinkles will return unless they have been separately treated with skin resurfacing: laser, peel, dermabrasion, or other techniques that are discussed elsewhere.

The face-lift operation can cause numbness in front of the ears and in the neck because tiny nerve endings are cut when the skin is lifted from the subcutaneous tissues. The amount of time it takes to regain normal feeling varies. Some patients may notice return of sensation within several days or weeks, but others will notice abnormal sensation for several months. Persistent numbness after several months is most unusual because the nerve endings should regrow into the skin.

As with any operative procedure, there are potential risks and complications that may require treatment. Fortunately, these complications are quite infrequent. If an untoward problem or a disappointing result does occur, honest and open discussions between patient and doctor are of paramount importance.

Complications

Hematoma

Hematoma is a collection of blood underneath the skin flaps that were lifted during surgery. It is prevented by meticulously stopping bleeding during surgery and by using a compressive facial dressing after the surgery. A drainage tube can help remove oozing blood, but it does not prevent all hematomas. The incidence of hematoma is more frequent in men than in women, probably because there are more blood vessels in the bearded male face than in the female face.

Despite good technique, a collection of blood may become large enough to require a second operation to drain (evacuate) the blood. This complication is most often caused by a rise in blood pressure that occurs as sedation and local anesthesia dissipate: the higher pressure can disrupt previously formed clots. A large hematoma that is not drained can cause healing problems and unacceptable scarring, which in turn can compromise final appearance.

Hair Loss and Hairline Disruption

Ideally, incisions in the hair are hidden in a good location, but even the best of techniques can cause a loss of hair next to the incisions. The incisions in the hair at the temples and in the scalp behind the ear must be meticulously planned, executed, and closed to reduce injury to the hair follicles. In most instances, the follicle is only "shocked," and hair loss is temporary; the hair should regrow.

Permanent injury to the hair follicles, which causes permanent hair loss at the incision, can occur if the skin that is lifted during surgery is stressed and not receiving adequate blood flow and, therefore, oxygen. If hair fails to regrow, the damaged area can be removed and reclosed; hair transplantation is another option (see hair chapter).

To avoid distorting the hairlines in the temple and in the scalp behind the ear, very careful planning determines the depth of the cut into the skin and the amount of excess skin to remove.

Skin Loss

After any operation where skin is lifted off the blood supply that lies below it, the skin can die; this potential complication is called necrosis, or sloughing of skin. Although it is infrequent, skin necrosis is an unusual but recognized complication of face-lift that occurs most frequently behind the ears and much more so in those with a history of tobacco use.

The chance of skin loss is minimized by avoiding excessive tension on the incision closure and by reducing risk factors and complications such as hematoma, infection, and cigarette smoking. It is for this reason that a patient must have a real willingness to avoid smoking for several weeks before and after the face-lift.

If an area of skin loss does occur, it will usually be treated with topical antibiotics and incision care rather than with another surgery. In many instances, the scars can be improved with local remedies such as applying silicone sheets or injecting cortisone. Once the incisions have completely healed and matured for several months, surgically revising the scars may be appropriate.

Infection

The face has a robust blood supply, so infection is a very rare complication after face-lift. Most infections that do occur are mild and can be treated with oral antibiotics. A collection of infected fluid or pus however would have to be surgically drained, which may compromise the final cosmetic result.

Nerve Injury

The most feared complication during a face-lift is injury to the facial nerve. The facial nerve supplies the muscles of expression. This nerve enters the face near the ear and has five branches—these branches control the vast majority of the movements of the face. Among the five branches of the facial nerve, the face-lift operation is most likely to injure the mandibular branch, a small branch to the muscles at the corner of the lower lip. Unless it is repaired, severing this nerve causes a permanent inability to lower the corner of the mouth. Fortunately, completely transecting (cross-cutting) this nerve happens infrequently. Weakness can occur after surgery if the nerve is bruised when the skin is lifted or the anesthetic agent is injected. Usually, nerve function will begin to recover after several weeks, although in some instances the nerve may remain weak for several months.

The other nerve branches that can be injured are the frontal branch, which lifts the eyebrows; the zygomatic branch, which closes the eyelids; and the buccal branch, which moves the upper lip. Again, permanent injury is very rare. If one of these nerves is damaged, it may recover function anyway. If it fails to recover, it should be repaired within the first year after surgery.

The greater auricular nerve provides feeling, or sensation, on the lower portion of the ear and earlobe. This sensory nerve is the most vulnerable to injury during a face-lift. If numbness is experienced after the operation, it should resolve within several months. Transecting the nerve is rare, but irreversibly cutting or injuring it may cause permanent numbness of the lower ear and earlobe. Attempts can be made at repair but typically are not as the remaining nerves tend to compensate over time.

The patient must understand that unavoidable but temporary numbness on the side of the face occurs. When the skin of the face is elevated and tightened, many tiny nerve endings in the facial skin must be cut. These small nerve endings regrow, restoring sensation to the overlying skin. The time it takes nerves to regrow depends on surgical technique and differences among patients. It may last weeks to months.

Scars

The scars after a face-lift should be barely perceptible. On occasion, however, scars may widen or thicken. This is most likely after a complication such as skin loss or delayed incision healing or when excessive tension is placed on the incision closure. Unfortunately, excessive scarring can occur without any specific cause in some patients, especially in those who are prone to keloids or hypertrophic scars, which are more common in patients with darker skin. If scars do thicken, scar creams, silicone pressure sheeting, or cortisone injections can reduce the inflammation of the scar, just as they do in treating skin loss. Any revision surgery to improve the scar should be delayed for at least three to six months—this will allow the scar to mature and surrounding skin to relax, making necessary revisions clearer.

Altered Pigmentation

A face-lift can create areas of skin that are lighter or darker than the patient's normal skin color, depending on location. Surgical scars may have less pigmentation than normal skin does if the cells that produce pigment (melanocytes) are stressed from the surgery. This may cause the face-lift incisions to show. On the other hand, skin can look darker if it contains old deposits of an iron-rich blood cell compound called hemosiderin. This hyperpigmentation usually resolves within six to eight months.

Ear Distortion

Tension on the ear, especially on the earlobe, can distort the normal ear shape. Neck tension can pull the earlobe down and attached to the neck skin, creating the "pixie ear," which carries the stigma of a postsurgical look: an earlobe that is pulled down. If this unusual attachment occurs, it can be corrected several months after the face-lift.

Facial rejuvenation is a wonderful operation that can take a decade or more off the face. The next chapter discusses adjunctive, or alternative, options for facial rejuvenation.

ADJUNCTS FOR THE AGING FACE: CHEEK AND NECK AND ALTERNATIVE PROCEDURES

Midface Lift and Cheek Restoration

In contemporary society, prominent cheekbones are considered an attractive attribute. Many patients who wish to have facial rejuvenation note the apparent descent of the "cheek." The traditional face-lift will lift the jowls, neck, and cheek skin between the cheekbones and ears. However, it does not lift the skin and tissues lying over the cheekbones themselves.

The major change in the midface (malar region) is the descent of a defined fat pad from the cheekbone. This tissue, known as the malar fat pad, contains dense, thickened fat and fibers and lies between the cheekbone (zygoma) and the nasolabial fold. It is just one of many soft tissues of the midface: skin, subcutaneous fat, and muscles. With aging, the zygomatic ligaments that support this pad stretch, allowing the fat pad to descend. This reduces the prominence of the cheek and deepens the crease at the nasolabial fold.

The other important component in the appearance of the midface is the cheekbone. As the malar fat pad and soft tissues sag below the most prominent part of the cheekbone, reabsorption of cheekbones can exaggerate the appearance of a long, thin face (see figure 17 again).

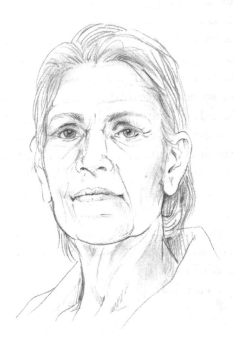

Figure 17

Midface Lift

In order to rejuvenate the midface, it is necessary to elevate the malar fat pad and to achieve a long-lasting improvement of the nasolabial fold. Aging in the midface is usually addressed at the time of a traditional face-lift procedure, but some patients feel that the neck and lower face are acceptably attractive. In this case, the midface lift may be done as an isolated procedure or in conjunction with an operation to rejuvenate the lower eyelids. The midface lift is a technically exacting operation that must be done by a surgeon who is well experienced in the technique.

Technique

The midface lift can be done under general anesthesia or under local anesthesia with intravenous sedation. This outpatient operation adds about an hour of surgical time to a lower face-lift.

The malar fat pad is exposed through one of multiple approaches: lower-eyelid incision, face-lift incision, incision inside the mouth, or endoscopic approach. Depending on the amount of desired elevation, the pad may be elevated by suspending it with superficial sutures. If a different elevation is desired, a deep dissection is carried out over the cheekbone and maxilla so that the muscles of the midface, malar fat pad, and overlying skin are elevated off the bone. This deep dissection may cause prolonged swelling, as described later in the "Alternative Face-Lift Procedures" section, particularly in "Subperiosteal Face-Lift."

After these midface soft tissues have been mobilized, sutures are used to suspend the tissues to a stable structure, usually the periosteum over the bone or fascia around the muscles next to the eye socket or in the strong muscular fascia of the temple. Tension should not be placed on skin. Careful attention must be paid to resuspending the lower eyelid to avoid placing excessive traction (pulling) on it. This added technique does correct the sagging malar fat pad, but critics have pointed out that there can be prolonged swelling over the cheekbone area that takes months to resolve. See figure 23.

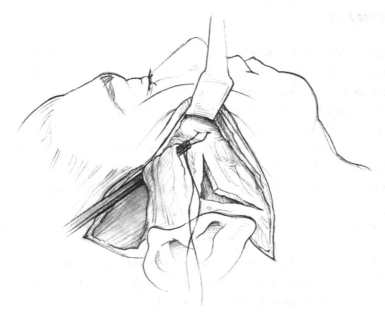

Figure 23: Midface LIft

Cheekbone Restoration

The majority of changes caused by sagging soft tissue can be treated with a midface lift. If, however, augmentation of the cheekbones is desired or preferred, malar implants may be inserted alone or during a traditional face-lift.

Many different types of implants have been described for malar augmentation. These materials are the same as those discussed in "Minimally Invasive Procedures," but the most commonly used material, by far, is a solid silicone implant. The implants come in a number of different sizes and shapes, making preoperative evaluation and planning extremely important. An excessively large implant can create excessive prominence of the cheekbones, causing a sunken appearance to the eyes. Small implants may lead to inadequate improvement.

Technique

Placement of an implant can be accomplished as an outpatient procedure with local anesthesia and sedation. Implants can be placed through one of three approaches. The most common approach, if inserting a malar implant is the only procedure being performed, is through an incision inside the mouth at the junction of the upper gums and upper lip. The implant can also be placed through an eyelid incision, which may be the approach of choice if a lower-lid operation (blepharoplasty) is done at the same time. The implant can also be placed through a face-lift approach when malar augmentation is combined with a face-lift procedure.

Healing

Tenderness, bruising, and swelling will occur in the malar areas in the initial postsurgical days. The pain should be readily controlled with oral pain medication. The bruising and swelling will resolve after several days, although it will be six to eight weeks before the final contour of the cheekbones is evident. In order to minimize swelling, ice should be applied frequently to the cheekbone area for the initial forty-eight hours, sleeping should be done in an upright position, and a light compression dressing may be used.

If the implant was placed through an incision inside the mouth, absorbable sutures that last several weeks will have been used. If the implant was placed through an eyelid or face-lift approach, stitches will be removed between a week, according to the surgeon's routine.

Complications

The biggest concern with malar implants is a poor aesthetic result. If the implants are not perfectly positioned, a noticeable lack of symmetry between the two sides of the face may exist. If the implant becomes displaced, a visible or a palpable implant will show asymmetry with the opposite side. If fluid or blood collects around the implant, it may need to be surgically drained.

Infections are rare and are characterized by pain, swelling, redness, and occasionally, drainage of pus through the wound. Mild infections may respond to antibiotics, but more severe infections may require removal of the implant.

Extrusion is a potential risk with any implant or other foreign body. If migration, trauma, or infection causes the implant to become displaced through the wound, the implant will need to be removed and replaced at a subsequent operation.

A large nerve called the infraorbital nerve descends along the cheekbone and supplies sensation to the side of the nose, upper lip, and middle teeth. If this nerve is injured or stretched during surgical dissection, temporary or permanent numbness can exist in these areas. In very rare instances, the implant will gradually migrate and push against the nerve, causing pain and the need for subsequent repositioning or removal of the implant.

Neck Lift

Changes in neck appearance are caused by (1) excess fatty deposits in the area below the chin and above the Adam's apple; (2) loose, hanging skin; (3) separation of the platysma muscle fibers along the midline of the neck; and (4) shortening and thickening of the edges of the platysma muscle, which causes vertical bands to form in the neck. With age, the platysma loses its attachment to the neck, so the natural tendency of muscle to contract and to shorten occurs. As a result, the junction between the chin and the neck loses its angle and appears blunted.

Technique with Face-Lift

The traditional face-lift will help address age-related problems in the neck, and is supplemented with the neck lift as an important part of a full face-lift. The elevation and tightening of the skin and SMAS in the face-lift operation will tighten the platysma muscle and skin of the neck, improving the contour of the neck-jaw angle. It restores the youthful appearance of the neck and reduces or eliminates the need for skin removal in the neck.

Any excessive fat in the neck, particularly beneath the chin, can be removed by neck liposuction, which can be done from the incision near the ears. However, enough other changes are usually needed in the neck that a $1\frac{1}{2}$" to 2" incision is made in the neck just below the chin. This new incision provides direct exposure to remove excess fat, address the muscles of the neck, and remove excess skin.

The platysma muscle often separates in front of the neck, causing a depression. In these cases, the two edges of the muscle are sewn together in the midline of the neck to provide a sling-like tightening of the neck; this technique is known as a platysmal plication. A back-cut is typically made to allow full tightening of the muscle in the midline and to disrupt the thickened vertical bands running down the neck. See figure 24.

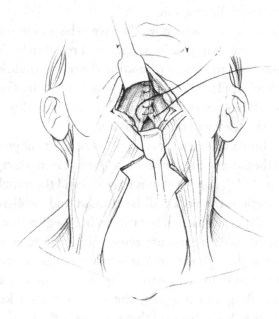

Figure 24: Neck Platysmal plication

These thickened bands can be treated with Botox, but the drug's effects are only temporary. As the face-lift is closed, tightening of the SMAS and tension behind the ear and along the posterior hairline will rejuvenate the neck.

Technique without Face-Lift

The sagging or fatty neck can also be improved by operations limited to the neck, which avoids a complete face-lift if it is not required or desired by the patient. If the neck deformity is caused only by fat deposits, liposuction alone may suffice. A small incision is made in the neck beneath the chin, and the fat is suctioned until a smooth contour is achieved.

Liposuction is not adequate if there is loose or hanging skin. In fact, the removal of fat can increase the sag of the skin if there is poor skin tone. This can be reduced with skin-tightening technology using external lasers or laser or ultrasound-assisted liposuction.

A slight excess of skin in the neck can be removed by excision through a horizontal incision high on the neck, just below the jawbone. The resulting scar should be fairly well hidden. This procedure may be done in conjunction with neck liposuction.

If there is a lot of loose skin, it would have to be removed through both horizontal and vertical skin excisions. This will result in both a transverse scar high on the neck and a scar extending down the middle of the neck toward the Adam's apple, which can be quite noticeable. For this reason, most surgeons will recommend removing excessive skin through a face-lift incision, where the scars will be well hidden.

Operations limited to the neck are typically outpatient procedures done with local anesthesia and sedation. Procedures last from thirty minutes for liposuction alone to $1^{1}/_{2}$ hours if skin is removed and the muscle is repaired.

After liposuction, the neck will be bruised and swollen. It may feel tight and even a little constricted, but this feeling begins to subside within seven to ten days. Neck sutures are removed in five to seven days. The patient will feel as through the neck is subtly swollen for several months. It can take up to two to three months to appreciate the actual result.

To limit swelling and bruising, the patient should keep the head elevated and wear either a dressing that surrounds the head and neck or a chin strap that compresses the swelling. Dressings will be removed in one to two days, but a chin strap is helpful for several weeks. If wearing the strap interferes with returning to activities and work, it is still recommended that the patient wear it at night and at other tolerable times.

If there is any lumpiness to the neck, daily massage helps disrupt fluid collections, limit scar formation, and reduce swelling. Massage therapy is designed to reduce fluid in the tissues and scarring. The discoloration of bruising will gradually resolve and descend to the chest because of the effects of gravity.

Alternative Face-Lift Procedures

Explaining the Terms

Other face-lift techniques do exist, and their names can be quite confusing to the public. It is the opinion of the authors and most other plastic surgeons that success is not determined by the exact technique chosen but, rather, by the ability of the surgeon to apply and modify his or her preferred technique to each patient's unique anatomy. That being said, clarifying of the "marketing terms" that exist is necessary.

Short-Scar Face-Lifts

The term "short-scar face-lifts" collectively refers to techniques designed to have shorter scars than a traditional face-lift. This can be easy in a patient who only needs a limited or mini face-lift. In addition, there is a group of techniques that seeks to avoid having to make an incision in the area behind the ear using applied physics. The reason for this is that the area behind the ear has no hair to mask any scarring that may occur. However, *the scar behind the ear is typically difficult to see because the ear and scalp mask the scar.* The incision in front of the ear is almost always required and typically heals very well, often being imperceptible.

Mini Face-Lift

A mini face-lift is essentially the removal of a limited amount of skin in front of the ear. The extended incision is not necessary. The deep support structures (SMAS) typically are not tightened with this technique. Some nice improvement can be obtained in early facial aging (wrinkles, folds, jowls), but it is not a dramatic change. As expected, the scarring and downtime are minimal. This procedure is typical of patients seeking some facial rejuvenation in their forties and can easily be done under local anesthesia. This is the basis for the Lifestyle Lift, a company recently declaring bankruptcy, but this proprietary lift has been modified in many ways over the years.

Lunchtime Lifts

"Lunchtime lifts" are quite different from face-lifts. These techniques use permanent sutures to catch the skin at key points and attach it to the fascia that covers the temporalis muscle at the temples. Skin excision is not made. The soft tissues underneath the skin are not lifted, and the effects are short-lived, typically two to five years. The presence of permanent sutures increases the risks of infection, exposure, scarring, and visibility; further, removing them is difficult.

"Weekend" Lifts

The "weekend face-lift" refers to a procedure to correct the loose skin in the neck. An incision is made beneath the chin, and excess fat is liposuctioned. The muscle bands in the platysma are removed and the muscle edges are pulled together in the midline with stitches. The inside of the neck is then treated with the resurfacing laser. Proponents believe that the laser tightens the skin, resulting in an improved neck lift. Skeptics believe that the benefit of a neck lift results from the traditional techniques of liposuction and repair of the muscle bands and that the laser treatment is of dubious benefit.

MACS Lift

The most common full face-lift but short-scar type of technique is a minimal-access cranial suspension (or MACS) lift. It is important to match the correct patient with this technique as a limited amount of skin is removed. This technique has been refined by many surgeons, and good results can be obtained.

MACS lifts use sutures in a single loop or a series of loops to tighten the face in several directions in the cheek region. The suture loops elevate the neck, tighten the cheek, and support the face. The fundamental support of the face from loop sutures anchored from several points in the lower cheek (a "multivector" technique) is strong and efficacious. After suspension of the deep structure, the skin is redraped and closed. The physics of this approach allow scars to be shorter than a traditional face-lift. This suspension technique can be combined with the traditional face-lift technique to augment rejuvenation.

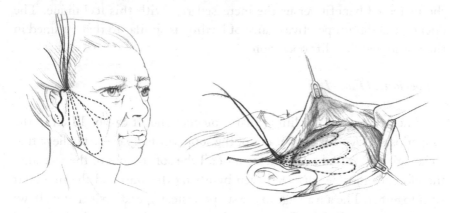

Figures 25 and 26 MACS Loop sutures

Composite Face-Lift

The philosophy of those advocating the composite face-lift is that gravity has an effect on all the soft tissues of the face, so lifting the skin alone is not adequate. The composite face-lift uses the same incisions described for the traditional face-lift procedure, but the dissection is carried out at a deeper level. The skin is left attached to the underlying orbicularis, SMAS, and platysma muscles.

Proponents of the operation have demonstrated some improvements over the traditional face-lift operation. Composite procedure restores the fat overlying the prominent area of the cheekbone in the mid portion of the face to a more youthful position. As the soft tissue of the midface is elevated, there is less overhang of skin at the crease at the nasolabial fold. Thus, the cheek can achieve a much nicer correction than is seen in the standard face-lift operation. The skin has more blood vessels because it is left attached to the deeper tissues below it. This may offer some advantage to the patients with a smoking history, who are at high risk for skin death.

This is a technically exacting operation, so it is imperative that the surgeon is experienced with the composite technique. The surgeon must work very carefully at this deeper level because the major branches of the facial nerve, which control facial expression, can be encountered. These facial-nerve branches could be injured by a surgeon who is not familiar with the details of this technique. The dissection is more tedious, and the operation may take an hour or two longer than a more traditional face-lift does. The decision to do a composite face-lift hinges on weighing the increased benefit versus the increased risk with this technique. The operative and postoperative course of healing is similar to that outlined in the traditional face-lift operation.

Subperiosteal Face-Lift

The periosteum is a lining that protects bone. It can be lifted in the subperiosteal face-lift. Advocates of the subperiosteal face-lift believe that facial aging is caused by the descent of all the soft tissues of the face and, therefore, cannot be corrected even by lifting the skin and the muscular layer together. The advantage of the subperiosteal operation is that it allows repositioning of all the soft tissues of the face, most importantly the fat pad over the cheekbone prominence of the midface. The subperiosteal face-lift is generally carried out in conjunction with a brow lift. The subperiosteal face-lift can be accomplished by lifting two levels of tissue in an "open" technique or by using an endoscopic technique, described below.

The subperiosteal face-lift combines two levels of dissection. The skin is elevated as described in the traditional face-lift operation. Then a second flap is created by using a technique to lift the periosteum, with the overlying muscles and fat, just above the bone. This is accomplished through incisions in the mouth at the junction of the upper lip and gum. This midface dissection carried out from inside the mouth is then connected to the brow-lift dissection. This frees up all the muscles and deeper tissues so that they can be lifted to their more youthful locations and sutured into position.

If the subperiosteal dissection (the layer lifted with the bone lining) is carried out during an open face-lift, sutures are placed from the superficial muscle layer to the fascia lining of the temporalis muscle under the temple skin. If the subperiosteal dissection is being done with an endoscopic technique, the suture is placed instead in the deep layers, not the superficial layers, of the muscle and then sewn to the same temporalis fascia.

As in the standard or composite face-lift, this is an outpatient procedure with similar anesthesia. The skin incisions are also similar but add the incisions inside the mouth. Because of the added subperiosteal dissection, the operation will take an hour or two longer than a traditional face-lift.

Proponents of this operation feel that it is safer and easier than the composite face-lift because the deep dissection is carried out beneath the facial muscles—just above the lining of the bone, where there are no branches of the facial nerve. However, the infraorbital nerve, which provides sensation of the midface, upper lip, and upper teeth, is vulnerable in the subperiosteal face-lift. The surgeon must carefully visualize and spare this sensory nerve during the dissection. If the patient later experiences any numbness to the lip, side of the nose, or upper teeth, the numbness should be temporary, disappearing within weeks or months but may not.

The biggest disadvantage of the deep-plane, subperiosteal approach is the much greater amount of swelling it causes than the traditional face-lift operation does. Swelling also lasts longer, as long as six months to a year.

Endoscopic Face-Lift

Endoscopic techniques have rapidly gained favor in surgery. The techniques that orthopedic surgeons use in arthroscopic joint correction are most well known to the public, and this technology has now been extended to a number of cosmetic procedures.

The endoscope is a narrow, tubular telescope that can be inserted into an operative site through a very small incision. The endoscope carries a small video camera and a fiberoptic light source; the image it creates is transmitted to a television monitor next to the patient or surgeon. Instruments can be inserted through these small incisions to dissect, trim, and remove soft tissues, as well as to place sutures. The surgeon visualizes and manipulates the anatomical structures with specialized instruments while viewing the video monitor. This enables an extensive operation to be accomplished through small incisions.

The endoscopic technique is not useful use for traditional face-lifts because the need to remove large amounts of skin necessitates lengthy incisions in front of and behind the ears. The technique, however, is very beneficial for extended procedures such as the subperiosteal face-lift and the forehead-brow lift.

THE FOREHEAD AND EYEBROWS

The forehead-brow lift operation is designed to correct sagging eyebrows, lift heavy brow skin that hoods the upper eyelids, and correct the deep wrinkles between the eyes and on the forehead. The forehead-brow lift operation can be carried out alone, at the time of a correction of the aging eyelids, or in conjunction with any of the previously discussed face-lift procedures.

The forehead-brow lift is an important part of facial rejuvenation in most individuals over the age of fifty. It can also be very beneficial in younger patients who have congenital or early descent of the brows. It may also be an essential component of operations to correct the upper eyelids: a significant number of upper-lid complaints may be caused by heavy brow skin that has descended onto the upper eyelid, a problem that cannot be corrected by surgery on the upper lids alone.

Eyebrow Position

In Western society, the most beautiful female eyebrow is considered one that begins near the nose at the level of the bony rim around the eye and arches to its highest point a few millimeters beyond the pupil. This highest point is about one centimeter above the bony rim. In men, the brow ideally lies along the bony rim throughout its length (see figure s 15 - 20

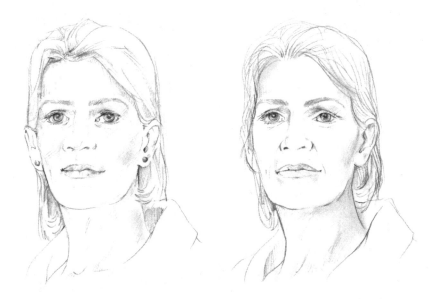

Figure 15   Figure 16

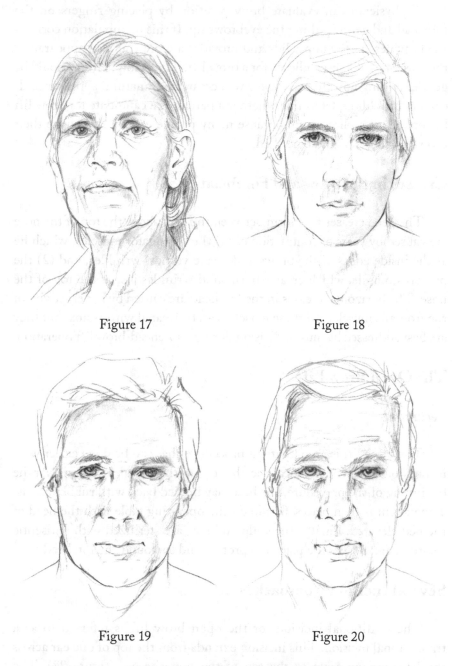

Figure 17

Figure 18

Figure 19

Figure 20

**Figures 15 and 18. Illustrations showing desired brow positions
in women and men with 16 and 17 showing progressive aging
in a woman and 19-20 showing progression in a man**

A physician can evaluate brow position by placing fingers on the forehead and gently pulling the eyebrows up. If this manipulation corrects the heaviness in the upper lids and provides a more youthful appearance, the patient is a likely candidate for a brow lift. The manipulation should be gentle: pulling upward excessively will create an unnatural appearance. It can be difficult to determine whether a patient is a candidate for brow lift by looking at a photograph because many people reflexively elevate their brows when being photographed.

Creases in the Brow and Forehead

The deep creases that form between the eyes above the top of the nose are caused by years of contraction of (1) the corrugator muscles, which lie at the inside edges of the brows and create vertical wrinkles, and (2) the procerus muscle, which creates horizontal wrinkles just at the top of the nose. The horizontal creases in the forehead are caused by hyperactivity of the frontalis muscle. All these muscles can be treated with Botox, but they are best addressed by muscle division during a forehead-brow lift operation.

The Open Brow Lift

Technique

The brow lift is an outpatient procedure that can be done either with intravenous sedation and local anesthetic or with general anesthesia. At the beginning of the procedure, the hair may be tied back with rubber bands. The patient is then placed faceup on the operating table with the head of the bed elevated. Finally, the scalp and face are sterilized with antiseptic solution, and drapes are placed to protect and surround the forehead.

Several Incision Approaches

The traditional incision for the open brow lift is referred to as a transcoronal incision. This incision extends from the top of one ear across the hair-bearing scalp to the top of the opposite ear (figure 27). The forehead lift is often carried out in conjunction with the face-lift procedure.

In this situation, the incisions are designed to join with the standard incisions of the face-lift operation.

The advantage of the transcoronal approach is that the scar will be entirely hidden in the hair-bearing scalp. The disadvantage is that the hairline will be lifted and rotated backward by the operation, elevating it half again (150%) as much as the brow itself is elevated. In other words, if the eyebrow is to be moved up by $^1/_2$ cm, the hairline will be moved up by $^3/_4$ cm. In most women with a normal hairline, this is not a problem. In men with thinning hair and in patients of either gender who have high foreheads, this traditional incision is not ideal because the hairline will be moved back even farther.

Figure 27. Illustration of patient's head showing the open-brow-lift incision

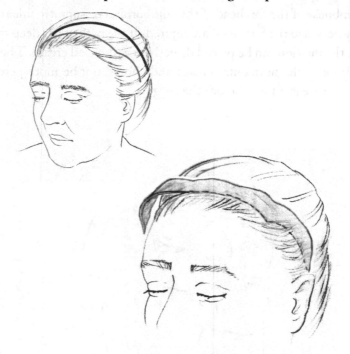

Therefore, the traditional incision can be modified to place the central portion of the incision at the junction of the hair-bearing scalp and forehead skin. This hairline incision is placed at the junction of the hair and forehead throughout its length. The incision is then taken back into the scalp at each temple, where the hairline is usually stable. Finally, the incision continues down to the top of each ear. This technique can be advantageous because the hairline is not moved backward, and in fact, in individuals with a high forehead, it can often be used to lower the hairline. The disadvantage is that there is a fine scar that may be visible, especially if the patient later wears the hair back or suffers hair loss. This incision is, therefore, most ideal in patients who have a high forehead and who are prepared to let their hair fall forward or wear bangs after the lift procedure. This is often not problematic because most women with high foreheads tend to avoid hairstyles where the hair is pulled tightly back.

In men with significant hairline recession or frank baldness, the incisions should be modified to make them less visible. One alternative is the excision (removal) of skin above the eyebrows, although this approach risks creating both a visible scar along the top portion of the eyebrow and numbness of the forehead if the supraorbital or supratrochlear nerves (sensory nerves to the forehead) are injured. If the patient has deep forehead creases, the incision can be placed directly in a forehead crease. The healed scar will lie in the horizontal crease and should not be more perceptible than the crease itself was before the surgery.

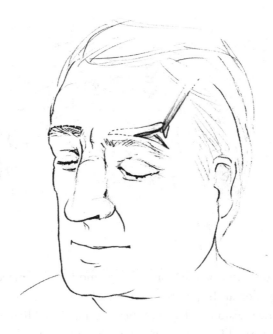

Figure 28. Direct brow lift

An increasingly popular technique is a mini brow lift, which uses a partial scalp incision. Typically, this incision is in the outer part of each brow and is wide enough to allow for elevation of the attachments of the brow to the bone, removal of undesired muscle, and limited removal of skin. The length of incision is less than the one used in a traditional standard open approach but greater than the one used in the endoscopic approach, described below. Specialized instruments are not required, so the surgical time is shorter than that needed in the endoscopic technique.

Correcting and Repositioning the Forehead

After the incision is made by one of the previously discussed approaches, the dissection is continued either below the subcutaneous fat layer or deeper, where the muscles of the forehead meet the periosteum (lining) of the frontal (forehead) bone. These layers are separated to just above the bony orbits (rims around the eyes), the upper eyelids, and the top of the nose. At that point, the dissection is deepened to travel along the bone itself, below the periosteum. The corrugator and procerus muscles are identified and almost completely removed; this step should permanently correct the wrinkles above the nose. Horizontal strips of frontalis muscle are removed to minimize recurrence of the forehead creases.

The forehead flap is then redraped, and the surgeon places traction on the scalp and forehead flap to determine the ideal positioning of the eyebrows. Excess scalp tissue is then removed so that, when the incision is closed, the wrinkles and creases will have been smoothed and the brows will have been repositioned. If a scalp incision has been made, the incisions are typically closed with staples. If a hairline incision has been used, forehead skin is removed and stitches placed at the junction of the forehead skin and hairline. The open forehead lift takes between one and two hours to complete.

The Endoscopic Forehead Lift

The objectives, patient preparation, and operative experience for endoscopic surgery are much like those outlined for the open technique. The endoscopic technique is appropriate for most people, but the incision location may need to be modified for patients with receding hairlines. Patients with elongated or convex foreheads should not use the endoscopic forehead lift. The major differences between open and endoscopic surgery are the length of the scars and tools the surgeon must use.

After sedation and use of local anesthetic agents, between three and five one-inch incisions are made in the scalp to allow the endoscope and specialized, endoscopic dissection instruments to be inserted, the forehead skin and muscle are lifted off the underlying bone. After the corrugator and procerus muscles are identified, these muscles are nearly completely removed. Horizontal strips of frontalis muscle are again removed under the forehead creases.

No scalp or forehead skin is removed with the endoscopic operation. The eyebrows can be repositioned internally with absorbable tines or with sutures that are fastened to absorbable screws or run through tunnels in the outer layer of the skull bone. Alternately, external, temporary screws may be fixed in the scalp just behind the hairline. The incisions in the scalp are closed with sutures or staples. Regardless of fixation method, the result is a brow lift where the forehead is elevated and pulled back: it readheres in the higher position allowed by the temporary fixation. The endoscopic brow lift usually takes between one and two hours to complete (see figure 29).

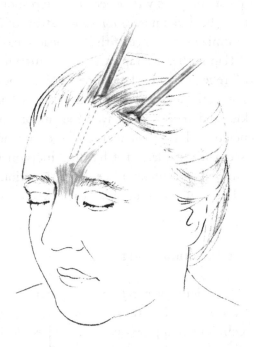

Figure 29. Illustration of the endoscopic brow lift

Recovery

After an open or endoscopic brow lift is completed, the head is usually wrapped with a mildly compressing dressing. This can be removed within twenty-four to forty-eight hours, at which point it is safe to gently wash the hair. Using ice and elevating the head for several days, especially during sleep, are necessary to minimize swelling after surgery. Occasionally, a suction drain will be placed for several days to limit any accumulation of fluid or blood. Pain and discomfort is usually minimal to moderate and is readily controlled with prescribed pain medication.

The amount of swelling and bruising experienced varies among individuals. Generally, the swelling begins to resolve after three to four days and should not be perceptible to others after a week to ten days. It is common to develop a fair amount of bruising around the eyelids, especially when the eyelids are part of the operation, because gravity causes forehead bruising to descend and eyelid skin is quite lax. In certain patients, both bruising and swelling may extend into the midface.

Sutures in a hairline incision are usually removed after one week. The stitches or staples, higher in the scalp, are usually removed by the end of the second week after surgery. If temporary external screws were used, screw removal after two weeks is a quick and painless office procedure that takes just a few minutes. The reabsorbable devices used with endoscopic technique may be palpable until they reabsorb after three to twelve months.

A patient should limit activities for the first week after surgery to minimize swelling and the risks of bleeding or disrupting closure or elevation. Nonstrenuous activities can be resumed at seven to ten days. Strenuous activity is limited according to the surgeon's judgment, typically for at least three to four weeks.

Complications

Risks and complications, while minimal, include hematoma, infection, long-lasting thinning of the hair around the suture lines, and prolonged scalp numbness.

A significant risk of making incisions in the scalp is a thinning of the hair near the incision. This is more common with a transcoronal incision than with the hairline incision because the tension that lifts the skin is held by the sutures that close the skin. The resulting stress on the hair follicles causes this hair-thinning; it is almost always temporary. It can take up to three months for the hair to regrow. In most instances, hair regrowth begins within several weeks. The scar itself will not typically regrow hair. This can make a transcoronal incision visible when looking.

Patients may initially experience an annoying numbness of the forehead and scalp; itching sensations also occur. With an endoscopic or transcoronal approach, elevating the brow and forehead places traction (pulling) on the nerves. This generally begins to subside after several weeks but may last for six months or longer.

With lower incisions (those above the brow, in a forehead crease, or in a hairline incision), branches of nerve fibers must be cut during the procedure. The numbness or tingling this creates above the incision can be quite severe initially; it may take up to a year for sensation to return as nerve endings regrow. The lower toward the brow the incision was made, the more likely this numbness is to occur.

Injury to motor nerves is extremely unlikely. Should injury occur, it is most likely to affect the vulnerable frontal branch of the facial nerve near each temple. This nerve allows the forehead muscle to move, so its injury would lead to both loss of animation of the forehead and early resagging of the brow on the injured side. An injury to the frontal branch is usually caused by bruising and stretching rather than by cutting. In these cases, the weakness is temporary. Support procedures or devices may be necessary while the patient waits for the reanimation of the forehead. Alternatively, the frontalis on the opposite side could be weakened with botulinum toxin type A.

THE EYELIDS

Eyelid surgery can help resolve the typical complaints of heavy or droopy upper lids, bags and puffiness of the lower lids, or excess, wrinkled skin in the lower lids. A natural consequence of aging, these characteristics can also occur prematurely in younger individuals. Bags and puffiness in the lower lids can occur even in the late twenties if there is a family predisposition to them. Heavy, hanging skin in the upper lids begins in some individuals in their early thirties. Many individuals complain of inappropriately looking tired, angry, or sad.

Female

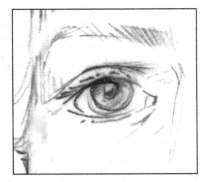 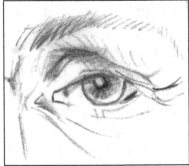

Male

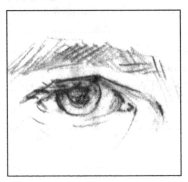 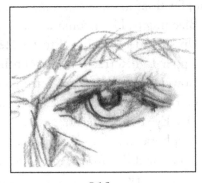

Younger   **Older**

Figure 30. Image of aged eyes

Blepharoplasty surgery, in simplistic terms, seeks to remove the excess skin and fat bags from the eyelids, either upper or lower. The changes that occur with age in the eyelids are a result of excess skin and protrusion of fat, but other structures may be involved or may even be the root of the problem.

Underneath the skin of the eyelids, the orbicularis oculi muscle covers a rim of cartilage known as the tarsal plate. It also covers the orbital septum, a layer of fascia (muscle lining) that is normally tight, behind which rests the periorbital fat (fat around the eyes). As aging weakens the orbital septum and stretches the orbicularis muscle, fatty tissue begins to protrude, creating the appearance of bags and pouches even when no excess of periorbital fat is present. In younger patients, there may be little or no extra skin, and all lid changes may be because of this protrusion of fat.

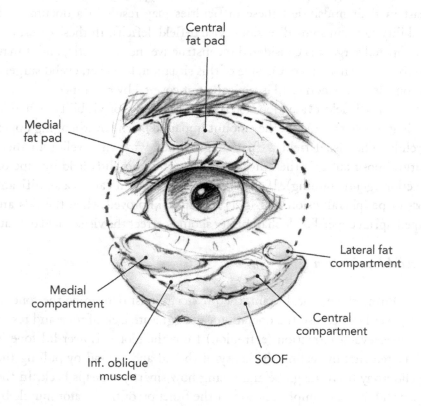

Figure 31. Eyelid fat compartments

Deciding Whether Surgery Is Appropriate

At the consultation, the anatomic changes in the eyelids and any contributing factors will be discussed in detail. In addition to assessing the skin, muscle, septum, and fat, it is important to appreciate any sagging of the eyebrows. This can be a major cause of upper-lid heaviness and wrinkling. The operation will tighten the skin and remove some of the heavy wrinkles. The lines and wrinkles next to the eyelids, the crow's feet, are not improved by the blepharoplasty operation.

Upper-Lid Vision Evaluation

In elderly patients, drooping of the upper-lid skin can actually interfere with vision on gazing upward and sideways. Typically seen in patients at least in their midsixties, these difficulties may result in a documented inability to see in some directions (visual-field deficit). In these cases, the anticipated surgery is considered reconstructive, not cosmetic, and it may be covered by insurance. Outside of this situation, however, eyelid surgery is considered cosmetic and is typically not covered by insurance.

A visual-field evaluation determines the scope of visibility (where a patient is able to see) and the amount impaired by the overhanging upper eyelids. The visual field is first diagrammed with the eyelids in their natural position. It is then diagrammed with the eyelids held by tape or traction (gentle pulling). If the excess upper-lid skin causes a significant loss of peripheral vision that is significantly improved when the lids are taped up, an upper-lid blepharoplasty should correct the visual field deficit.

Eyelid Evaluation

During the physical exam, the physician must determine the tone of the lower lids because the operation can aggravate lack of tone and result in lower-eyelid retraction (ectropion) from the globe. Lower-lid tone is evaluated first by feeling the laxity of the lid and second by pulling the eyelid away from the globe and seeing how smartly it snaps back. In the upper lid, it is also important to test the function of the levator muscle by measuring the position of the eyelid margin with extreme upward and downward gazes. The levator muscle in the upper lid is responsible for opening the upper lid and holding it in a normal position sitting at the junction of the colored and the white portion of the eye. If the levator shows poor function and is not corrected, upper-lid ptosis (drooping) will occur after surgery. Patients with environmental allergies that cause episodes of swelling, especially in the lower lids, will continue to experience similar allergy symptoms after the surgery.

General Health and Eye Health

Medical conditions are important variables in determining the safety of eyelid surgery and the type of anesthesia to be used. The physician must be made aware of any chronic illnesses such as high blood pressure, diabetes, heart disease, and certain thyroid problems (hyperthyroidism or hypothyroidism).

Evaluation before surgery also includes a discussion of any problems with the eyes, such as a change in visual acuity, cataracts, glaucoma, or any history of dry eye as blepharoplasty can aggravate these processes. A simple test to gauge tear production, a Schirmer's test, may be performed. For this slightly uncomfortable test, filter paper is held against the globe (eyeball) for several minutes; the volume of tears produced is then measured. For severe eye diseases, a preoperative consultation with, or clearance from, an ophthalmologist may be necessary.

The Blepharoplasty Operation

Surgery on the eyelids may be done as an isolated operation or in conjunction with a face-lift, brow lift, or other procedure. Both upper and lower eyelids can be corrected at the same operative setting; alternately, one pair of eyelids can be corrected as an isolated procedure. The procedure is almost always performed around both eyes.

Blepharoplasty is an outpatient procedure that is typically done with intravenous sedation and local anesthesia. Some surgeons prefer to have a patient remain awake. Certain procedures, especially in the upper eyelids, can be done with local anesthesia in the office. However, lower-eyelid surgery and more invasive techniques may require deeper anesthesia.

Surgery for each set of lids takes about forty-five minutes to one hour, and the surgery on all four lids lasts $1 \frac{1}{2}$ to 2 hours. If all four lids are being operated upon, most surgeons will perform the upper-lid operation first. Patients typically go home shortly after the sedation has worn off.

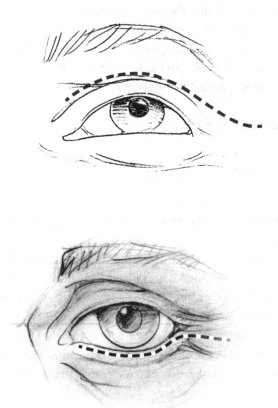

Figure 32. Typical skin incisions for eyelid surgery

Upper-Eyelid Surgery

The main goals of an upper-eyelid blepharoplasty are to remove excess skin and muscle and correct protruding orbital fat

Patients will be positioned either sitting or lying faceup, and after adequate sedation or anesthesia is established, the face and eyes are cleansed with an antiseptic solution. The eyelids are marked carefully after determining the anticipated effect; the marked skin is then excised to remove hanging skin and provide a youthful appearance.

After skin removal, a strip of orbicularis oculi muscle is then removed to create a new supratarsal fold (the fold that runs along the upper eyelid, also known as the superior palpebral fold). A small incision is made in the orbital septum (fascia layer) to provide access to the two fat compartments of the upper lid. Excess fat behind the orbital septum is then teased out and removed. Prominence at the sides of the upper eyelid may be caused by an enlarged or hanging lacrimal tear gland, which should not be resected but can be elevated and resecured.

The levator muscle may need to be shortened or plicated. Any bleeding is controlled with an electrical device that coagulates the bleeding points. The incision is then closed with small sutures. Most surgeons prefer to use a running, continuous stitch located just beneath the surface of the skin, typically with the ends of the sutures held in place with adhesive tape.

Lower-Eyelid Surgery

Lower-lid blepharoplasty is also designed to remove excess skin and to correct the bags and puffiness caused by fat protrusion (see figure XVI-3). The amount of skin removed is usually very little because aging occurs to a greater extent in the deeper structures, namely in the orbicularis oculi muscle and three fat compartments, in the lower lid. Excess skin resection leads to ectropion, eyelid retraction with a less protected globe that is both unsafe and unappealing.

The lower-lid blepharoplasty may be done through a multitude of techniques. A skin incision is used if both skin and fat are to be removed. If only fat is to be removed or corrected, the procedure may be done through an incision on the inside of the eyelid, a transconjunctival blepharoplasty. Laser surgery is also available.

As with the upper-eyelid operation, patients will sit or lie faceup before being given adequate sedation or anesthesia. Then, the face and eyes will be cleansed with an antiseptic solution.

Technique with Skin Incision

With the skin approach, an incision is made one to two millimeters below the eyelashes; it extends into one of the creases on the side of the eyelid. The skin and muscle of the lower eyelid are dissected to expose the underlying orbital septum (fascia). A small incision is made in the orbital septum, and the prominent fat lying behind the orbital septum is identified. This fat is either removed or redistributed over the bony orbital rim and in the tear-trough deformity, where it is usually sutured into its new position with absorbable sutures. Redistribution of the fat can prevent or correct a hollowed, periorbital appearance of aging.

Once the fat excess has been corrected, a limited amount of excess skin and muscle is removed from the skin flap. If the patient has festoons (herniation of the orbicularis oculi muscle), the protruding muscle is trimmed. If there is any laxity in the lower eyelid, a suspension procedure will be done. Most commonly, a stitch below the skin is used to tighten or resecure the ligament in the lower eyelid to the bony rim on the side of the eye (procedures known as canthopexy and canthoplasty, respectively). These steps prevent laxity of the lid, eversion of the lid away from the globe, or actual retraction of the lid (ectropion). Finally, the incision is closed with very fine stitches.

Technique with Incision Inside the Eyelid

In a transconjunctival blepharoplasty, the incision is made along the inside lining (conjunctiva) of the eyelid. Once the conjunctiva has been incised, the septum and fat compartments are identified and excess fat can be manipulated or removed until the puffiness in the lower lids has been corrected. The primary disadvantages of this technique are the inability to remove excess skin, the limited ability to redistribute fat, and the inability to resuspend the canthal ligament. However, the lack of an external scar is an advantage. Further, it is safe to use the resurfacing laser or chemical peels to treat fine wrinkles in the skin because skin is not elevated in this alternative approach. Septal reset, or tightening of the fat compartment, can still be performed.

Technique with Laser

Some surgeons prefer to use a laser technique for the blepharoplasty procedure. Typically, a cutting CO_2 laser is used to make the incision. The procedures are essentially the same as those outlined for upper- and lower-lid blepharoplasty. However, the cutting is done with a laser rather than with knife and scissors. Proponents of laser blepharoplasty believe that there is less oozing and, therefore, less bruising and swelling after surgery.

Recovery

The most common complaints after blepharoplasty are oozing, crusting, swelling, bruising, dry eye, and pain. The pain or discomfort that develops as anesthesia wears off can be readily controlled with prescribed medication. Oozing and crusting may occur but can be limited with good care. After any form of blepharoplasty, using ice packs or ice-soaked gauze and elevating the head for the first forty-eight to seventy-two hours will help minimize swelling.

Bruising and swelling will develop within several hours of the procedure and usually peak at forty-eight to seventy-two hours. After surgery on all four eyelids, lids may swell to cause almost complete closure of the eyes. Usually by the fifth day, swelling will have resolved significantly. Bruising is variable, peaking anywhere between several days to a week after surgery. Resolution can be quite rapid over another several days, but it may take up to ten to fourteen days to resolve.

Postoperative symptoms of dry eye are usually temporary and can be managed with lubricating gel and eye drops. Contacts should not be worn until the swelling and dryness have resolved. Symptoms of blurry vision, light sensitivity, or tearing may occur but should slowly resolve over two to three weeks.

Sutures are removed four to seven days after surgery. Once the stitches are out and the swelling has subsided, makeup can be used to cover up any residual bruising. The scars will be red and noticeable in the initial weeks before they slowly begin to fade. It may take up to three months for the scars to settle down fully. During this time, incisions should be protected from the sun as much as possible to encourage scars to heal more beautifully. Once the scars have fully resolved, they should be barely perceptible.

The return time to work and other daily activities is variable: some patients return as quickly as five days after surgery, while others may not feel comfortable getting back to work and going out in public for weeks. Strenuous activity should be avoided for three to four weeks after surgery in order to minimize swelling, bruising, and the chances of bleeding.

Complications

Complications are rare, and most individuals can expect an excellent result with correction of their eyelid problems. There are, however, potential risks and complications.

Bleeding or Hematoma

Bleeding below the skin may require the surgeon to reopen the incision (explore the incision) and coagulate any bleeding areas. Superficial hematomas that are left undrained increase scarring and alter the appearance of skin after recovery.

Severe bleeding behind the eye (retrobulbar hematoma) can lead to blindness. It causes severe pain, visual changes with loss of visual field or bright lights and sparkles, proptosis (protrusion of the eyeball), or excessive bruising and swelling. This is an emergency that requires immediate release of sutures and the ligament that holds the cartilage around the eye.

Upper-Lid Drooping (Ptosis)

In most instances, upper-eyelid ptosis (drooping) after surgery results from swelling in the upper-lid muscles and resolves as the swelling improves. In rare instances, the levator muscle or Mueller's muscle, both of which lie behind the orbital septum (fascia layer) and elevate the upper lid, may have had poor function that was not detected before surgery or may have experienced injury or bleeding. If ptosis persists after swelling has resolved, it may require reexploration and repair of the levator muscle.

Upper-Lid Retraction (Lagophthalmos)

The skin excision done in an upper-lid blepharoplasty is designed to create enough tension on the eyelid that it may be difficult to fully close the eyes for a few days after the operation. However, if an excessive amount of skin has been removed—especially in conjunction with a brow lift—a patient may lose the ability to close the upper lids. If the cornea of the eye is exposed during sleep, the resulting risk for corneal ulceration and permanent damage must be prevented with lubrication gel at night to protect the cornea. If this problem fails to resolve, surgical correction and even skin grafting may be necessary.

Lower-Lid Retraction (Ectropion) and Inversion (Entropion)

Ectropion, pulling of the eyelid away from the globe, is avoided in most instances by carefully preplanning the amount of skin to be removed from the lower eyelid. Even after removing an appropriate amount of skin, severe lower-lid swelling and bruising can occasionally pull the lid down or away from the globe. This is best treated prophylactically with tape or a Steri-Strip to hold the lid in a normal position for several weeks during the early recovery phase. This helps avoid a longer-lasting lid retraction from developing as scar tissue forms. A longer period of taping will correct the problem even in most difficult cases.

If excessive skin is removed from the lower lid, the lid margin will be pulled down by the tight closure. Even if no skin or the correct amount of skin has been removed, ectropion can also result in a lid with poor tone. This complication can be avoided in most instances if the poor tone has been identified before surgery (see "Lower-Lid Evaluation," above) and the lower-lid cartilage is suspended at the time of surgery with a canthoplasty or canthopexy. If surgery was done with a transconjunctival approach, the patient may suffer an entropion, which draws the eyelid inward and may cause the eyelashes to irritate the cornea.

If an ectropion or entropion persists for three months or longer, surgical correction is likely necessary. These are difficult, exacting operations that must be done by a surgeon who is well-versed in the techniques of repairing ectropion and entropion.

Corneal Abrasion

As mentioned above, corneal injuries can cause discomfort and damage to the eye. Corneal abrasions (scratches) can occur during surgery (that is, from use of a surgical sponge) or from corneal exposure (that is, from lagophthalmos or ectropion). They can be confirmed with fluorescein dye and a Wood's lamp examination. Treatment requires antibiotic therapy and lubricating eye ointment.

Dry Eye Syndrome

Dry eyes are characterized by itching, scratching, burning, light sensitivity, and discomfort. Swelling and crusting after surgery is temporary in most cases and is managed with lubrication and artificial teardrops. In rare instances, a prolonged or permanent dry eye syndrome may occur, even when preoperative evaluation showed normal tearing (Schirmer test).

In such cases, drops and medications to increase tear production may be effective.

Epiphora

Excessive tear production is usually caused by eye irritation but may be caused by disrupted drainage from the lacrimal tear duct. The Jones dye test can determine if drainage is normal. If it is, then simple symptomatic treatment of excessive tearing is appropriate. If it is not, the surgeon must determine whether swelling has caused limited drainage or whether surgical repair is necessary.

Continued Prominence of Lids

Any of the five fat compartments in the upper and lower lids may be inadequately corrected. This problem may be addressed after swelling resolves and it is determined which one or more fat compartments are the culprits. It is important to remember that the fat compartment of the upper eyelid that is farther from the nose contains the lacrimal (tear) gland, which should not be resected but can be sutured higher to the orbital rim. Weak orbicularis oculi muscles may need additional tightening, especially in patients who had festoons (herniations of orbicularis muscle) before surgery.

Asymmetry

As with any procedure on matching features of the body, attaining symmetry is more than half of the battle. Any asymmetry across the eyes can be obvious and may require surgical revision.

Residual Wrinkles

Lower-lid blepharoplasty will not remove all the fine wrinkles on the lower lid. Because removing too much skin from the lower lids can risk ectropion after surgery, the surgeon may have chosen to leave a small amount of residual, lower-lid, excess skin. After a sufficient recovery period of several months, this can be corrected or improved with excision of additional skin or with skin resurfacing using a chemical peel or laser.

THE NOSE

The nose is the most dominant feature of the face. Serving as the center and the most forward feature in profile, it is always on display. Therefore, dissatisfaction with the nose has always been one of the most common reasons to seek plastic-surgery consultation. The operation to reshape or recontour the nose is known as a rhinoplasty; *rhinos* is the Greek word for *nose*. The procedure was popularized in Europe in the late 1800s and has been slowly refined over the years.

A multitude of techniques now exists for correction of both the aesthetic appearance and the function of the nose. The operation is technically difficult, but gaining the insight required to determine what needs to be done to any given nose to meet a patient's expectations is significantly more difficult. Of all the plastic-surgery procedures, rhinoplasty results are the most variable. Good results require both experienced physician judgment and skillful technique, so it is important to select a surgeon with interest and experience in rhinoplasty.

The structures of the nose are pyramidal in shape, and the operations to alter the shape of the nose are directed at sculpting of the bone and cartilage framework. The draping of skin over a framework of bone and cartilage determines the nose's contour. The skin also contributes to the overall shape and appearance of the nose. Unfortunately, little, if anything, can be done to change the skin. The thinner and smoother an individual's skin is, the better the nose can be reshaped: the skin will redrape better over the refined bone and cartilage. Thick, oily skin will not redrape as well and will negatively affect the final result. The skin of the nose tends to be thicker and oilier at the nasal tip, and it gradually thins as it ascends the nasal dorsum. There is a wide variability in skin characteristics among different races, sexes, and individuals.

Evaluation of the Nose for Surgery

The evaluation of the nose, even more than with any other procedure, is a dialogue between patient and surgeon. It is important that the patient shares likes, dislikes, and goals, as well as what is perceived in the nose and what change is desired. The plastic surgeon should explain how the patient's wishes translate to what anatomy will need to be worked on and, especially, what can and cannot be accomplished. Patients are always concerned about how the nose will look after surgery. Results can be difficult to convey even with the advances of digital photography and computerized image "morphing." These technologies can be helpful, but they cannot and should not be expected to serve as crystal balls. It is most important that the surgeon verbalizes what he or she sees and intends to change, as well as a general idea of what can be expected. A patient should not have confidence in a surgeon who cannot put such ideas into words that are clearly understood.

There are important external landmarks that must be analyzed and discussed in order to clarify the intent of surgery and the patient's cosmetic expectations

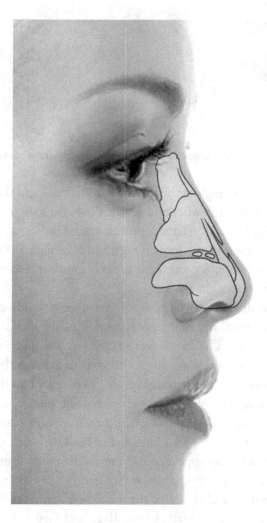

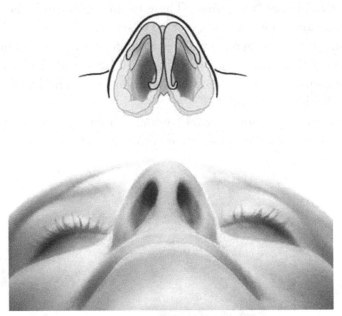

Figures 33 and 34. Images of internal nasal support structures

- The nasofrontal angle is the junction of the nose and the forehead. The area at the top of the nose is called the root (radix) of the nose. It may be ideally shaped, prominent, or deficient. A deficient nasofrontal angle is not deep enough and can create the appearance of a humped nose. A prominent radix is too deep and will enlarge the appearance of the nose.
- The nasal dorsum is the roof of the nose extending from the forehead to nasal tip. The upper portion of the roof is shaped by the nasal bones. The two bones on the left and right meet at the roof of the nose and slope down the sides to meet the bones of the face. This portion of the nose is rigid. The lower two thirds of the nose are comprised of cartilage—this part of the nose is malleable. Seen from the side in profile, the nasal dorsum may be ideally shaped, prominent (as in a humped or hooked nose), or deficient (causing a ski-jump appearance). Viewed from the front, the nasal dorsum may be ideally shaped, too narrow, or too wide, depending on the position and slopes of the nasal bones and cartilage.
- The supra-tip area is made of cartilage and forms the roof of the nose just above the nasal tip. The supra-tip area will usually have

170

the same characteristics as the roof of the nose, but there may be an isolated deformity, especially in those who have had disappointing results from previous surgery.

- The nasal tip is an obvious feature. Its appearance is determined by the tip cartilages. The nasal tip may be ideally shaped, too sharply pointed, too rectangular, too square or boxy, too round, or too prominent. It may also not project enough.

- The columella is the base of the nose between the nostrils; it connects the tip of the nose and the upper lip. Its junction with the tip defines the tip-columella angle, while its junction with the lip defines the nasolabial angle. The nasolabial angle is ideally 90° to 100° in men; in women, it is slightly more shallow, 100° to 110°.

- The nasal lobule (or nasal ala) is the soft, flared portion of the nose that forms the roof of the nostrils on each side, extending from the nasal tip to the cheeks. The edge is called the alar rim. The lobule may be ideally shaped, too thick, or too thin, or it may hang too low, lift too high, or flare too much.

The nose must be evaluated with regard to the underlying facial anatomy. In seeking a change, an individual must be aware that the area of concern may be a problem of perspective caused by the underlying facial skeleton. A perceived hump may, in fact, be a small hump that looks big because of a small chin. A projecting tip may only appear to project because the upper jaw is prominent. A long nose may be balancing a long midface, so excessive nasal shortening would provide an unacceptable result.

Physiology of the Nose

Of course, the nose not only serves as a focal point for beauty and appearance but also serves the important physiologic function of breathing. It filters dirt or particles out of the air, humidifies the air before it reaches the lungs, brings the temperature of breathed air closer to body temperature, and protects the air. Abnormal anatomy may cause difficulty breathing by reducing the area of the passage, whether it is comprised of fixed anatomy or functional obstruction.

The vomer is the bone on which the cartilage of the septum sits. The turbinates are structures of bone, cartilage, and mucous membranes that occupy the side of each nasal passage. The nasal septum is cartilage lined by mucous membranes and ideally lies exactly in the middle of the nose between the two air passages. If it is displaced off the midline or if there are spurs off of the septum, one or both airways may be limited. The vomer and turbinates exist to enlarge the surface area available for the important functions of the nose, but if they are too large or project and obstruct the airway, the resistance to the passage of air becomes too great.

Two functional valves in the nose exist to regulate this resistance. The external nasal valve is the front edge of each nostril and is shaped by the alar rim, the columella between the nostrils, and the floor of the nose. The internal nasal valve is formed higher, inside the nose between the septum, the nasal floor, and the upper outside cartilages of the nose. If either of these valves is narrowed after previous trauma, infection, or surgery, a functional septorhinoplasty is appropriate. Correction of the nose internally for breathing purposes and externally for cosmetic purposes can be done at the same time.

Rhinoplasty Surgery

Nasal surgery is usually not considered until a patient has completed the adolescent growth spurt, usually after sixteen years of age in boys and fourteen years of age in girls. Surgery can be performed on a child or a young adolescent if it is limited to the nasal tip only. However, in our opinion, extensive surgical procedures on the nasal septum, nasal bones, or cartilages can interfere with subsequent growth.

Even if no breathing problems exist before cosmetic rhinoplasty, a plastic surgeon may recognize that narrowing or otherwise changing the nose for cosmetic reasons may restrict nasal breathing in patients with borderline anatomy. In these cases, the surgeon should recommend surgically repairing the internal structures (such as a deviated septum, excessive turbinate size, and collapsed nasal valve).

Insurance Concerns

Cosmetic surgery on the nose is not covered by insurance, whereas surgery to correct functional problems typically is. However, health insurance does not cover functional problems that are caused by cosmetic surgery. Frequently, even when some functional problems are present before cosmetic surgery, health insurance still does not cover the cosmetic rhinoplasty. However, if a real need for surgery can be demonstrated, a portion of the combined procedure might be covered. Finally, reconstructive nasal surgery because of previous injury, surgery, or disease process also may be covered by insurance.

It is imperative that the patient and surgeon communicate with the insurance company before surgery to seek the guidelines for coverage and obtain preoperative approval if the operation or a portion of it is to be covered by insurance.

Technique

Rhinoplasty is usually performed as an outpatient procedure in the surgeon's office facility, in an outpatient operating room, or in the hospital. Most rhinoplasties can be performed under local anesthesia with intravenous sedation, but if more extensive procedures are anticipated, especially to address airway problems, the operation may be done under a general anesthetic. The operation will take between one and three hours.

There are two major rhinoplasty techniques, which are based on the degree of incision and exposure. The technique used depends upon both the extent of modifications planned and the surgeon's preference, as there are different schools of thought on the risk to benefit ratio of each.

In the closed technique, incisions are made inside the nose. The closed technique provides plenty of exposure to address the upper nose but limited exposure of the nasal tip.

In the open rhinoplasty technique, incisions are made through the inside of the nose and across the columella, which allows wide exposure to the entire nasal skeleton of bone and cartilage. If extensive work needs to be done on the nasal tip or if complex grafting is required, the added exposure from the open technique greatly outweighs the drawbacks of the minimal scar in the columella (see figure 35). The swelling after open-incision surgery is greater and longer-lasting.

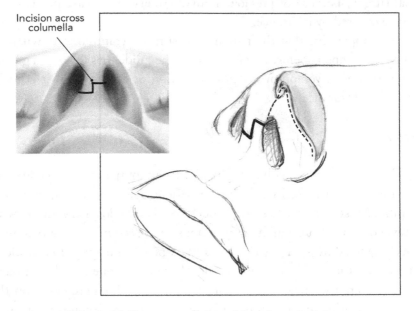

Incision across
columella

Figure 35. Diagram of open rhinoplasty incisions

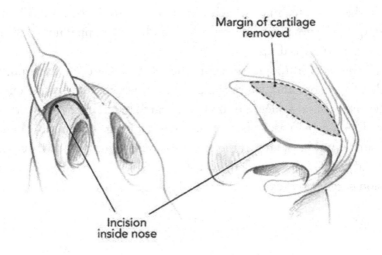

Margin of cartilage
removed

Incision
inside nose

Figure 36. Diagram of closed rhinoplasty incisions

The most common goals of the basic rhinoplasty include improving the appearance of the nasal tip, correcting the projection of the nasal dorsum, narrowing the bony skeleton, or shortening the nose.

The Tip

The tip shape and projection can be changed by sculpting any excessive tip cartilage, by suturing any tip cartilages that need to be repositioned, or by grafting carefully sculpted cartilage to fill in any deficiencies. Cartilage for grafts is typically taken from either the nasal septum or from behind the ear. The specific technique or combination of techniques is determined by the appearance of the tip and the desired change.

Nasal Dorsum

Excessive projection of the bridge of the nose gives the appearance of a nasal hump. When the abnormality is limited to the dorsum, it can be addressed by removing and filing the projecting nasal bones and upper nasal cartilages. If significant bone is removed, the pyramidal shape of the nose may be lost and become flat along the bridge, so the nasal bones may need to be precisely fractured to narrow the bones and recreate an angle in the midline. If the projection also includes the radix and extends from the forehead to the tip rather than there being an obvious hump, the appearance may be that of a "Roman nose." In this scenario, both areas may need to be addressed, but it is necessary to verify that the anomaly is not actually a deficiency of the tip.

On occasion, the appearance of a hump may be caused by a deficiency of bone at the nasofrontal angle and deficiency of cartilage at the tip instead of an excess of tissues in the nasal bridge. These situations actually require cartilage grafts to build up the radix and nasal tip.

A "deficient bridge," often referred to as a *saddle nose deformity*, is most commonly seen as a result of loss of cartilage resulting from previous surgery or injury to the nose. Patients who have a mild to moderate deficiency of the nasal bridge require augmentation, typically with a cartilage graft. In the case of severe deficiency, a larger graft is needed, and synthetic implants or bone may be used. Bone grafts may be harvested from the outside layer of the skull, the crest of the iliac bone above the hip, or the ribs.

A wide nose can be narrowed by infracturing the nasal bones at the junction with the maxillary bones and the face (at the side of the nose next to the cheek). The nasal bones are then moved inward to narrow the base and vault (breadth) of the nose bridge. This procedure is also done after removing a large bony hump to prevent the creation of a wide appearance at the bridge of the nose, as mentioned above.

Nasal Length

The skeleton of the nose determines the shape of the nose. A long nose can be shortened and moved upward by sculpting and removing extra cartilage and by shortening the lower portion of the nasal septum. It is important to carefully balance the length of the nose relative to the length of the face and to avoid creating a "pig snout," which can occur if the end of the nose is moved excessively.

The Crooked Nose

A nose may be crooked because of previous trauma or surgery or as a consequence of normal development. This condition is usually a result of having a crooked or displaced nasal septum. Straightening the nose usually requires both realignment of the deviated septum (septoplasty) and infracture of the nasal bones.

Nasal Flare

Excessive nasal lobule or alar flare can be corrected by removing a wedge from the lobules at the point where the nose connects to the lip or by removing a wedge from the bottom of the nostril just above the lip. Both techniques cause a barely visible scar.

Recovery

After the operation, the nose may be packed with absorbent material for twenty-four to forty-eight hours to limit bleeding. Overnight observation may be required to monitor postoperative bleeding and breathing if significant work inside the nose, such as septal reconstruction, or extensive external reconstruction is performed. Tape or skin Steri-Strips are used to compress the nose to try to limit swelling. If work has been done on the septum, temporary splints may be sewn inside the nose to keep it straight as it heals; these are usually removed within two weeks. If the nasal bones were infractured, an external splint is used to stabilize the bones as they heal for seven to ten days. If open rhinoplasty incisions were made, external stitches across the columella must be removed within a week to minimize scarring. Stitches inside the nose will dissolve on their own.

The nose will initially be tender and swollen after surgery. Depending on the amount of work done on the septum and bones, the eyes may also be bruised and swollen. By using ice to soothe the area around the eyes and nose for the first twenty-four hours after surgery and avoiding a fully reclined position, the extent of any swelling and bruising can be limited and will usually begin to resolve within seventy-two hours. However, in some cases, the bruising can last two weeks. Swelling is commonly worse in the morning or after any prolonged period of lying down. Therefore, patients should sleep in a semiupright position to minimize this swelling and bruising. Drainage around the nostrils occurs for several days and may be brightly blood-stained. Pain and discomfort is fairly easy to control with prescribed medication and begins to subside within several days. Most people are able to return to work, school, or daily activities while the external splint is in place. Once the splint is removed, tape or Steri-Strips may be kept on the nose for another week. Light exercise can be resumed within two to three weeks and strenuous exercise within four to six weeks.

It is quite natural for patients to be concerned about their appearance, but bruising, swelling, and external dressings used in the initial two weeks are temporary! As they resolve, subtle changes in the nose will begin to appear: patience is necessary as several more weeks are required to notice improvement. Some swelling will remain for several months, at which point significant improvement can be seen, but the final result may not be fully appreciated for up to one year after the operation.

Because the nose is such a prominent part of the face and defines appearance, some patients may be disappointed after rhinoplasty if their preoperative expectations are overly optimistic. This again emphasizes how important it is to have discussed fully what can and cannot be accomplished and what appearance should be expected during the various stages after surgery. Otherwise, even minor postoperative problems can cause significant anxiety.

Secondary or Revision Rhinoplasty

Revision rhinoplasty may be appropriate after a disappointing result. In most instances, it is wise to delay any revision for at least twelve months to allow all swelling to resolve and scar tissues to soften. Secondary rhinoplasties are even more technically difficult than the first nasal operation, and it is imperative that patients seek out a surgeon who is experienced in secondary rhinoplasty.

The surgical techniques are similar to those detailed in the section above on primary rhinoplasty surgery, but the anatomy is quite varied and difficult to discern. Most secondary rhinoplasties necessitate an open approach, even if the initial rhinoplasty was performed closed. This will improve the access to the nasal framework and allow for better appreciation of previous anatomy and changes made. Grafts are more frequently necessary in secondary revisions. Obviously, an innumerable number of problems may occur in a primary surgical procedure, but some of the more common deformities are correctable by revision. They include residual humps, the ski-jump deformity, the supratip deformity, and several types of tip deformities.

Residual Hump

A residual hump may remain when the bridge of the nose is not sufficiently corrected. Occasionally, even if the hump has been well-corrected, scar tissue can cause little spurs of bone and cartilage that produce a bump or prominence on the nose. These problems are easy to correct with a revision procedure to file down the area. The revision can usually be done through the small incision of a closed approach.

The Ski-Jump Deformity

If the surgeon removes too much of the cartilage and bone along the bridge of the nose when reducing a hump, the nose can have the appearance of a saddle or ski jump. This can be corrected by grafting cartilage, bone, or synthetic material in the deficient dorsum. Donor sites for the cartilage graft include the septum of the nose, the conchal bowl of the ear, and the cartilaginous portion of the rib. Donor sites for the bone include the iliac crest above the hip, the outer layer of the skull, and the ribs. Synthetic implants are continually being developed and evaluated.

Supratip Deformity

A supratip deformity refers to a lack of depression or dip between the nasal tip and the bridge of the nose, causing this area to be too flat. In severe cases, an elevation occurs. It is also known as the "polly beak" deformity because the nose has an appearance reminiscent of a parrot's beak. A number of very different problems may cause this deformity: (1) a buildup of scar tissue after an otherwise well-done rhinoplasty, (2) a surgeon's failure to remove the cartilage in the supratip area when correcting the bridge of the nose, or (3) excessive surgical correction of the nasal bridge above the supratip area, where too much cartilage in the tip of the nose was removed. The cause of the deformity must be determined to clarify which corrective measures are needed. Correction may include either (1) making the tip or bridge of the nose higher in profile by grafting cartilage or (2) making the supratip area lower by removing septal or nasal cartilage.

Tip Deformities

If the tip cartilages are reduced too much, the resulting loss of tip projection will require revision with cartilage grafts taken from the nasal septum or the ear. Scar tissue can distort the tip cartilages, thus requiring repositioning of the tip cartilages. Finally, undercorrection of a projecting tip may be revised with further sculpting of tip cartilage.

Pinched or Excessively Narrowed Nose

If too much cartilage is removed during the original rhinoplasty, there may be a pinched look to the nose. The narrowed nose may interfere with breathing and require correction with cartilage spreader grafts to improve appearance and open the internal nasal valve.

Nostril Deformity

Disappointing nostril results usually have asymmetrical nostrils, instead of a specific abnormality. Problems are usually caused by either asymmetry of the tip cartilages or scar tissue distorting the cartilage on the soft tissues of the nasal ala. Repositioning and resculpting the nasal-tip cartilages, with or without using cartilage grafts, can repair this situation.

Complications of Rhinoplasty

Bleeding

Bleeding often occurs in the initial days after surgery. If packs have been placed into the nostrils, bleeding will most commonly occur after pack removal. If bleeding occurs, it can usually be controlled with ice and light pressure, use of an inhaled vessel constrictor (such as Afrin nasal spray), and remaining calm in a sitting or somewhat upright position. On occasion, bleeding may require repacking of the nose. It rarely causes any true long-term effects, such as cartilage reabsorption or skin loss.

Infection

Infection is extremely unusual after rhinoplasty because a proficient blood supply protects the nose. But should it occur, infection is heralded by spreading redness from the incision and increasing pain and swelling. Packing and dressings can make it difficult to detect an infection. Minor infections respond to oral antibiotics.

Rarely, a severe infection can occur, especially if the nose is still packed. Packing left longer than a couple of days causes the risk of the patient developing toxic shock syndrome, a rare but serious disease caused by a toxin (the toxin is produced by staphylococcal or streptococcal bacteria). If a patient has a strong suspicion of a developing infection, it should be discussed with the physician immediately.

Failure to Improve Breathing

As mentioned, the airway can be modified to improve ventilation if preoperative evaluation suggests that doing so would be beneficial. However, there are medical conditions such as allergies, infections, irritants, or immune-system problems that may cause persistent difficulties with breathing.

THE LIPS

Modern, aesthetic ideals prefer a full lip, even bordering on pouty, but not too thick. Common complaints related to the lip include lips that are too fat, lips that are too thin, elongated lips that extend down to the level of the incisor (front) teeth, lips that are too short and show too much tooth, and lips with excessive wrinkling. Even those with ideal lips can expect the upper lip to become thinner and longer with advancing age. Lip wrinkles become progressively more prominent with age. The rate of wrinkling is greatly increased by sun exposure and cigarette smoking.

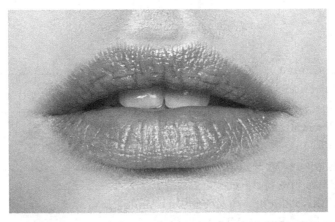

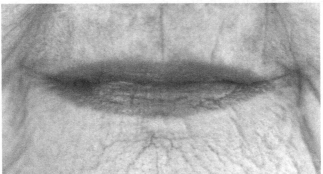

Figure 37. The aging lip

The upper lip lies between the nasolabial folds on each side of the face, and these folds form the junction between the upper lip and cheek. The outward-showing lip consists of skin on the upper part and the vermilion, which is the red mucosa that hangs free at the bottom of the lip. In the middle of the lip sits a depression, the philtral dimple, bordered on each side by the philtral columns that extend from the red mucosa to the nose.

The border between the red vermilion and skin is a fine white line known as the vermilion-cutaneous margin. The lower lip consists of (1) the free red vermilion with a less defined vermilion-cutaneous margin and (2) lip skin that extends to the crease at the junction with the chin.

Lip Enhancement

Lip Injection

Thin lips can be enhanced by a number of techniques that include (1) plumping by injecting collagen, fat, or other fillers, typically hyaluronic acids (i.e., Restylane, Belotero, or Juvéderm); (2) surgical placement of permanent or semipermanent implant material (ADM); or (3) surgical enhancement. Thin lips can be fattened by injecting manufactured fillers, collagen, or one's own body fat. Before deciding to inject a foreign material, it is imperative to carefully discuss the substance being injected.

There is a multitude of materials that can be injected, but the perfect filler is the Holy Grail of minimally invasive cosmetics right now. Many products will continue to be developed in this rapidly expanding field. An in-depth discussion of fillers can be found in the chapter "Minimally Invasive Procedures."

Injectable Fillers

Injecting fat removed from another area of the body has become quite popular. Sufficient experience around the country indicates that minimal, serious complications or health hazards after injecting fat occur, and no allergy testing is necessary because the fat is taken from the patient's own body. This technique does require preparing and manipulating the fat before transfer.

Numerous agents have rapidly been developed as fillers. There are permanent fillers, semipermanent fillers, and temporary fillers. The most popular fillers at present are based on hyaluronic acid, which is a natural product in the human body and, therefore, does not require allergy testing. Other products are synthetic or are developed from animals or cadaveric tissue.

Liquid silicone was a popular injectable filler in the past, but after a flurry of unverified reports linking connective tissue disorders and silicone products, the sources of injectable silicone are no longer provided by established companies. In addition, late effects of injected silicone show a propensity for migration, infection, extrusion, calcification, and distortion. Because of its risks and the multitude of safer options, injecting liquid silicone should be avoided.

Fillers, as mentioned, are of highly variable permanence. Injectable collagen, fat, and most fillers will be slowly reabsorbed. Collagen usually lasts about three to four months, so retreatment may be necessary three to four times per year to maintain effect. Occasionally, fat will be reabsorbed within several weeks, but in most instances, it lasts for three to four months and can last much longer.

Procedure and Recovery

Lip injections are performed on an outpatient basis. Anesthetic is typically not required, but ice or a topical anesthetic agent, such as EMLA, may be applied to the lip before injection. The collagen, filler, or fat is then injected into the lip until the desired fullness has been achieved. Depending on the product, overcorrection of the lip may be necessary to account for some immediate absorption of material. The lips will swell after injection, but the swelling should begin to subside within several days. The lip may feel tight and uncomfortable during this period, and bruising may occur.

The potential risks with any injectable agent may include infection, injury to structures, or embolism (injection of the implant that causes blockage). There have been very few serious long-term complications reported, but there are, however, common pitfalls. If the injectable material is not distributed evenly, areas of lumpiness can form. Even with an ideal distribution of fat, uneven, slow reabsorption can cause an irregular shape in the lip.

Lip Implants

Implant Types

The lips can be permanently plumped by inserting a solid implant rather than liquid. The implant material options, as discussed in the chapter "Minimally Invasive Procedures," are solid silicone, Gore-Tex, Medpor, or acellular dermal grafts. Silicone and Gore-Tex do carry risks—including extrusion, migration of the implant, and distortion of the implant—but they can be safely used in most circumstances. SoftForm is a tubular, Gore-Tex implant that is introduced into the lip by a patented injection apparatus that reduces contamination and eases the procedure. Medpor is porous, a beneficial feature that allows ingrowth of the patient's lip tissue, reducing migration and infection but making it difficult to remove or adjust the implant later. Acellular dermal grafts and autogenous tissue (dermis, fascia, and tendon) are much less prone to infection, scarring, and extrusion because they become incorporated into the body as host cells replace the product. However, they may ultimately be reabsorbed.

Procedure and Recovery

Most lip implants can be introduced in a short, outpatient procedure. The lip is numbed with a local anesthetic that blocks the nerves of the lips. A small incision is made at both corners of the lip. The implant is introduced through one incision, and the opposite side is used to position the implant. These two very small incisions are then closed with one or two stitches each. If a patient donates his or her own tissue, procedure time obviously increases, and the donor site must heal.

After the procedure is complete, the lips will be tender and swollen. This usually resolves within a week or two after the procedure. The implants can provide a permanent, aesthetic plumping of the lip, but as with any foreign body, there is the risk of complications. A mild infection may be treated with antibiotics. Any significant infection will require removal of the implant. Migration of the implant may distort the lip and ultimately lead to its extrusion or penetration through the skin: this requires removal of the implant.

Lip Enhancement—Surgical Technique

There are several surgical techniques common for shortening or enhancing the skin of the thin, elongating lip. The procedures may be either a lip procedure alone or part of a face-lift, a more extensive facial rejuvenation operation. In lip advancement, a small strip of skin is removed at the vermilion-cutaneous margin, the area of the lip where the skin meets the red mucosa (See figure 38). When this incision is closed, it gently pulls up the mucosa, providing a shorter, fuller-appearing lip. Because the excision lies along the entire length of the lip, both the central portion and corners of the lip will be corrected. The resulting scar is a fine white line that in most cases blends with the normal edge of the red part of the lip. However, the scar can be noticeable if it fails to blend at the junction.

In a lip lift, a small oval-shaped portion of skin is removed from the upper area of the upper lip at the junction with the nose. As the incision is closed, it lifts the lip, shortening it (see figure 38). The operation results in a scar; however, at the nose-lip junction, it is usually well-hidden and barely visible beneath the contour of the nose. The fact that this operation will not correct drooping of the lip at the corners of the mouth (the commissure) distresses many patients.

A **B**

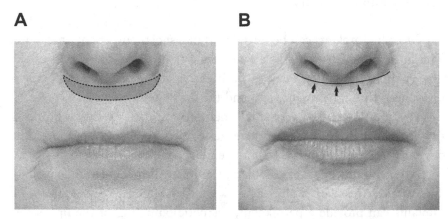

Figure 38. Diagram of lip lift

Plumping the lip can be surgically performed without implants by moving forward tissue from inside the mouth. This requires creating a series of flaps in the mucosa of the mouth, which are advanced toward the mouth opening. The plumping effects may diminish over time, but later implant or injection procedures are still available.

All the lip surgical procedures are performed as outpatient surgery under local anesthesia with a local anesthetic block to the nerves of the upper lip. After the operation, the lip will be tender and swollen. Any pain can be easily controlled with prescribed medication. Stitches are removed at approximately one week. Most of the bruising and swelling should resolve by a week after surgery and can be reduced by applying ice. Risks and complications are minimal, but they include bleeding and infection. Should either of these occur, treatment is readily available. The biggest concern with excising skin is the development of a visible scar.

Lip Reduction—Surgical Technique

Lip reduction is a procedure to reduce a prominent or protruding lip. It is an outpatient procedure done with a local anesthetic. It is easy to anesthetize the lip with either direct injection or a block of the nerves to the lips. The incision is made on the inside of the lip, where an oval-shaped strip of mucosa is removed (see figure 39). Depending on how the excision has been designed, closing the incision should either pull the lip in or shorten the lip. The procedure should take less than one hour and cause minimal discomfort after surgery. Typically, swelling takes three or four days to resolve significantly but could take up to ten days. The sutures used to close the incision are usually reabsorbable, but if the sutures are uncomfortable or the material is slow to dissolve, the sutures can be removed after six or seven days. Complications are minimal but include bleeding and infection, which would require treatment with antibiotics. Prophylactic antibiotics after surgery are frequently used because the mouth has a population of microorganisms. The greatest concern is that too much mucosa may be removed, which can lead to excessive shortening or asymmetry between the lips.

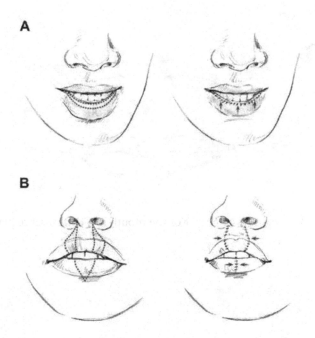

Figure 39. Diagram of excisions used in lip reduction

Corner of the Mouth Lift

Another useful procedure for the aging mouth is correction of the downturned corner of the mouth that gives the appearance of a permanent scowl. This can be done be excising in the nasolabial fold but a less visible scar is possible with an excision around the corner of the mouth, directly turning it up. The results of even a few millimeter change can be dramatic.

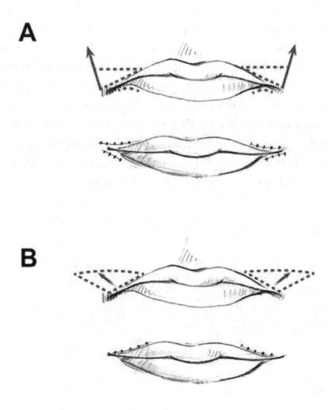

Figure 40. Diagram of corner of the mouth lift, commissure plasty

THE CHIN

The chin is the lowest portion of the central face and, as such, draws considerable attention. Anatomically, it extends from the crease below the lower lip to the first crease below the chin. This submental crease marks the beginning of the neck. The lateral borders of the chin are below the corners of the mouth, where the skin of the chin blends with the skin of the cheek.

Aside from ethnic variations in shape and projection, the ideal tip of the chin from a side, or profile, view lies along a line extending from the nasal tip to the lower lip, while the curve between the lip and chin should be in line with the curve between the nose and forehead. A chin positioned behind these points will look deficient, while a chin extending in front of these points will appear too far forward (prognathia).

Chin complaints are usually based on either vertical or forward dimensions. The aesthetics of the chin are determined not only by its shape and projection but also by the position and structures of the jaw, face, and neck. An unattractive chin may indeed protrude or be deficient as a result of an isolated chin deformity, but frequently, it will appear abnormal because of its relationship with other, less-than-ideal facial features, which must be addressed to achieve true correction. The relationship between the nasal profile and the chin profile is important. A deficient chin can make the nose look larger, while a large nasal hump may exaggerate the appearance of any chin deficiency. It is not uncommon for a plastic surgeon to recommend both a chin correction and a rhinoplasty if the chin is exacerbating the appearance of the nose or vice versa.

The Deficient or Small Chin

Augmentation of the Weak or Deficient Chin

Chin Implants

A mild degree of retrogenia (setback chin) or microgenia (deficient chin) can be corrected by a quick, relatively simple placement of a prosthetic chin implant. Placing an implant will provide an aesthetic correction of a mildly to moderately small or weak chin. It is not advised for severe retrogenia or chin deficiencies.

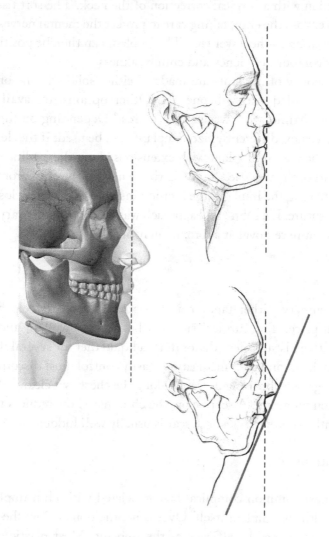

**Figure 41. Image of the severely deficient chin
on bottom versus the ideal on top**

The Procedure

Chin augmentation with implants can be performed as an outpatient procedure with local anesthesia and light sedation. The incision is typically made inside the mouth between the lower lip and the gum, but it can also be made in the submental skin immediately below the chin. This latter approach is more commonly used if the chin augmentation is being done

191

in conjunction with a surgical correction of the neck. The soft tissues are elevated to expose the chin, taking care to protect the mental nerves, which provide sensation to the lower face. The implant can then be positioned to correct the contour deficiency and chin weakness.

The majority of implants are made of either solid silicone or a solid silicone wall filled with silicone gel. Other options are available, as discussed in "Minimally Invasive Procedures." Depending on the degree of chin deficiency, differently sized implants can be used; if the deficiency extends to the jaw, an implant with extensions along the jawline can also correct some of the weakness of the jawbone next to the chin prominence. After positioning the implant, the incision inside the mouth is closed with absorbable suture. If a submental approach was used, the temporary sutures used will require removal at approximately one week.

Recovery

After surgery, either tape or a chin strap is used to help hold the implant in place. The surgical site will be tender, swollen, and mildly bruised. If there is sufficient discomfort, a liquid diet for several days may be beneficial, but oral pain medications easily control most discomfort. As healing progresses, bruising descends along the chest as it clears—bruising is not reason for alarm. A scar below the chin may show redness for three to six months before it fades; the scar is usually well hidden.

Complications

The most common complications associated with chin implants are problems with the implant itself. Over time, the bone below the implant may erode, reducing the efficacy of the implant. Most plastic surgeons minimize the risk of bony erosion by placing the implant above the periosteum, the soft tissue lining of the bone. Erosion can be particularly problematic if the implant has been placed too high on the chin overlying, the tooth roots.

If the implant is dislodged or migrates, it will cause an asymmetric correction of the chin or impinge on the mental nerve that provides sensation to the skin of the jaw. Correction requires surgical repositioning. A dislodged implant, very infrequently and usually as a result of an injury to the chin or an infection, may extrude through the incision, necessitating its removal. Infection is a rare complication but is heralded by pain, redness, and progressive swelling. Should the infection fail to respond to antibiotics, implant removal is again necessary. After implant removal either because of infection or extrusion, a new implant could be placed at a subsequent operation after the chin is fully healed, typically at least three months later.

Chin Advancement: Genioplasty

In more severely deficient or weak chins, correction is best accomplished with chin advancement, known as a genioplasty (see figure 42). This is a more complicated operation than a chin implant, but it is safe if it is done by a plastic surgeon who is adequately trained in advancement techniques. The surgical decision should be based on what the patient needs, not on any technical limitations of the physician, so all patients seeking chin correction should consult with a surgeon who has enough training and experience to be comfortable with both chin advancement and chin implantation techniques.

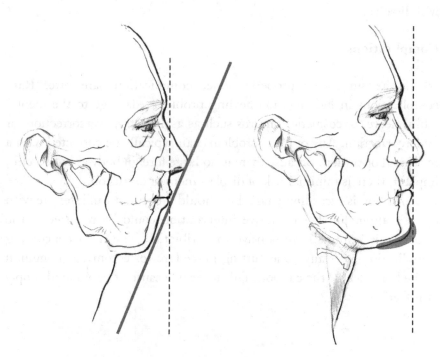

Figure 42. Image of the results of a genioplasty. Can be enhanced even further by a chin implant, as showed in gray.

The Procedure

Chin advancement can be done as outpatient surgery under either local anesthesia with appropriate sedation or general anesthesia. An incision is made between the lower lip and the gingiva, as in the placement of a chin implant. The tissues are dissected off the bone, again protecting the mental nerve. Using a special bone saw, the lowest portion of the chin is cut free and can then be moved. For a standard advancement, it is moved forward and held in position with plates and screws, called a sliding genioplasty. If more vertical height is necessary, the chin can be lowered; a bone graft may be required. This bone graft is typically harvested from the hip.

Recovery

After surgery, there will be pain, swelling, and bruising for longer than after a chin implant, but comfort should be easily attained with oral pain medication, and solid foods can usually be eaten within several days. A chin strap can protect and reduce swelling. The sutures inside the mouth will dissolve.

Complications

If the surgery is properly done, complications are rare. Rare complications include incision-healing problems, damage to the mental (chin) nerve, or cosmetic concerns such as asymmetry, overcorrection, or undercorrection. Any of these problems can typically be corrected with a revisional operation. Because there is no large foreign body as with a chin implant, there is minimal risk of displacement or extrusion.

Infection is exceedingly rare, but should it occur, it can interfere with bony healing. Further operative intervention could be required if the infection is minimally responsive to antibiotics. The most concerning complication after any bone-cutting procedure (osteotomy) is nonunion of the bone, where the cut bone fails to heal because of poor blood supply or infection.

The Protruding Chin: Chin Reduction Surgery

The Procedure

A chin that extends too far forward can be corrected by a chin reduction. If a deformity is caused by excess chin projection only, the operative approach is similar to that for chin advancement. An incision is made inside the mouth, and the soft tissues are elevated from the underlying chin.

Several steps may be taken, depending on each patient's needs:

❖ A mild increase in projection of the chin can be recontoured by burring down the excess bone on the front of the chin.

❖ A more significant protrusion may need to be set back by cutting the lower portion of the chin free from the remaining jaw and repositioning accordingly.

➢ If the chin simply projects too far, the segment is set back and maintained in position with wires or plates and screws.

➢ If the chin also needs shortening, a wedge of bone is removed between the chin and the lower teeth; this allows the chin to be reduced backward and upward.

➢ Any final contour discrepancies are finessed with a bur to provide a smooth appearance to the chin.

If only moderate bony changes are planned, this procedure can be done with local anesthesia and sedation. If more extensive bony work is required or a patient has low tolerance for surgery, general anesthesia may be preferred. In either case, reduction can be accomplished as an outpatient procedure.

Recovery

After surgery, there will be moderate pain, swelling, and bruising. The pain should be readily controlled with pain medication and several days of a soft diet. Swelling will resolve slowly over several weeks. The contour will begin to be evident within seven to ten days, but the final result may not be evident for several months.

Complications

The most frequent complaints after this operation are related to disappointment with the aesthetic results. It is more technically challenging to provide the desired correction with a chin reduction than with a chin advancement. The soft tissues overlying the chin make estimating the effects of bony reduction difficult to estimate during surgery. If a significant reduction is carried out, the soft tissues may not redrape well, leaving some extra skin and soft tissue in the chin and jowl areas.

Other complications are similar to those stated above and include rare infections, incision-healing problems, and damage to the mental nerve. Should any of these occur, later surgeries may be needed.

The Poorly Positioned Upper and/or Lower Jaw

Preoperative evaluation by a properly trained surgeon is critical before performing any facial bone-altering surgery. There are circumstances when an unattractive chin may reflect a much larger problem with the facial bones, the mandible (jawbone), or the normal relationship in which the upper and lower teeth meet. An individual with an overdeveloped middle third of the face may have a long maxilla (upper jaw), which results in a down-and-in rotation of the chin. A poorly positioned lower jaw can also appear to retreat if the lower jaw is underdeveloped or is positioned back into the head. Conversely, a lower jaw that is overdeveloped or abnormally positioned forward from the head may manifest as a protrusive chin.

During consultation regarding the chin's appearance, a careful examination of other facial bones and the relationship of the upper and lower teeth (occlusion) is necessary. Radiographs or an orthodontic evaluation may be necessary. Significant maldevelopment or malpositioning of these structures is most appropriately corrected by maxillofacial surgery to reposition the abnormal upper jaw, lower jaw, or both. If surgery on the upper or lower jaw is needed but the surgeon attempts to camouflage the overall deformity by operating on the chin only, then a serious worsening of the overall appearance can result.

Soft-Tissue Concerns

The soft tissues of the chin may be a source of complaints for patients, either because of congenital characteristics or changes with age. The most common complaints are related to a lack of definition of the chin, but this pseudodeficiency may be due to excess skin or fat surrounding and/or below the chin.

The Double Chin

The appearance of a small chin is aggravated or caused by excess fat in the submental region, the portion of the neck immediately below the chin. This "double chin" is most commonly seen in individuals with a short neck that lacks a well-defined, sharply angulated junction between the horizontal portion of the neck below the jaw and the vertical neck. The loose, hanging skin drapes down over the trachea, esophagus, and other structures; it can mask chin projection, so correcting the neck may correct the appearance of the chin. Much of the information below is detailed more fully in the section "Neck Lift."

Liposuction

This correction may be minimally invasive in a younger individual with tighter skin and minimal to moderate excess fat. A simple liposuction of the excess fat below and behind the chin can allow the skin to redrape, causing it to adhere more tightly to the jawbone and neck and create a sharper cervicomental (neck-jaw) angle. However, the skin may have lost enough elasticity that it cannot tighten sufficiently without additional treatments that combine well with liposuction.

Lasers and Ultrasound

Some plastic surgeons advocate treating the inside surface of neck skin. Originally done with the carbon-dioxide resurfacing laser, a moderate amount of extra skin could contract, but the technique was difficult. This has been replaced by laser liposuction (i.e., SmartLipo), which offers a variety of wavelengths on the tip of a fine cannula that can be used to laser the fat and undersurface of the skin with a minimally invasive technique.

The laser energy leads to collagen and elastin renewal, thus correcting some of the loose skin in the double-chin area.

Another method of treatment is ultrasound-assisted liposuction (i.e., Vaser). Laser and ultrasonic liposuction technology allow controlled damage of the deepest layers of skin, leading to its later contraction. Both laser and ultrasound-assisted liposuction techniques are effective for mild to moderate skin excess.

Surgical Skin Lift

For more serious skin redundancy, actual excision of skin is necessary and may be referred to as a neck lift. If only a small amount of skin needs removal, a direct horizontal excision of the skin beneath the chin can be done, but this will result in a scar. It is important that the incision be made immediately below the jawbone to make the scar less visible.

Severe excess skin is best addressed through a lower face-lift approach, as discussed more fully in the "Face-Lift" and "Neck Lift" sections. Many patients who are unhappy with their necks are happy with their faces and feel that a face-lift approach is more surgery than they need or want. However, using a face-lift incision allows the surgeon to tighten the muscular layer that supports the neck and to remove skin in less visible areas (behind the ear and into the back hairline). All of the above are outpatient procedures that can be performed with local anesthesia and, as needed, sedation.

Jowls

Large jowls next to and obscuring the chin are more difficult to address locally. In certain cases, jowls may be addressed with liposuction. Local excision leaves conspicuous scars. The definitive way to address such jowls is with a face-lift.

The Chin Cleft

Much less frequently, a patient may be dissatisfied with the cleft of the chin, either feeling that it is too deep or too shallow. If the surgeon agrees with this self-assessment, the cleft can be surgically addressed.

A shallow cleft can be deepened with either direct removal of soft tissue or liposuction along the vertical midline of the chin. On rare occasion, the surgeon may approach the chin through the mouth, as discussed above, to remove some of the central bone with a bur.

An excessively deep chin cleft can be addressed with a chin implant, contoured to fill in the cleft more than the rest of the chin, or with burring of the prominent portions of the chin. Each of these techniques leads to significant swelling in relation to the amount of desired change, and the true effects may not be visible for months.

The Chin Lift

As the face ages, the chin and its fat pad also descend, creating a "droopy chin" or "witch's chin." Either alone or in conjunction with full facial rejuvenation, a chin lift is often needed. This is most often performed through an incision between the inside lower lip and gum, similar to the one discussed above. After freeing the soft tissues of the chin from the bone and the skin, a suture can suspend the chin to a fixed object, typically bone or its lining, the periosteum.

The Ears

A number of problems can occur in the development of the ear, which may lead to the need for corrective surgery, typically as a child but occasionally as an adult. The shape of the ears is determined by the development and growth of a cartilage framework over which thin skin tightly adheres. About 80% of ear growth has occurred by the time a child is five years of age, but surgery on the ears is usually delayed until the child is at least six years of age, at which point rib cartilage is adequately developed to use in reconstructing the ear. It is after this age that one's peers become more aware of unique physical differences, and childhood ridicule may begin.

The most common ear deformities for which one may seek correction are anotia (absent ear), microtia (small ear), constricted ears (cup ear, lop ear, and cryptotia), macrotia (large ears or prominent ears), otohematoma (cauliflower ear), or earlobe size/shape anomalies. These repairs are usually reconstructed in adolescence between the age of seven and ten. Alternatively, tissue molding may be completed in infancy, ideally in the first few months of life while the cartilage is still malleable due to the blood-born estrogen in the infant's system from the mother. This has always been very challenging but a new proprietary product has simplified the process (Earwell, Becon Medical Ltd, Naperville, Illinois). In contrast to other parts of the ear, the earlobe is especially prone to changes with age that may cause the elderly to seek cosmetic correction.

Anotia and Microtia: Small Ears

The small ear deformity is referred to as microtia and is caused by underdevelopment of the ear cartilages. The most extreme example of microtia is total absence of the ear. Both anotia and microtia require complex, multistaged reconstructions to mold the cartilaginous portion of the ear and provide it with durable skin that will adhere to the cartilage properly. The intricacies of the surgeon's technique are beyond the scope of this book, but the complete reconstruction of the ear is frequently divided into stages, but certain techniques are combined. Typically, the first stage uses synthetic implants or cartilage grafts to create the framework of the ear. Cartilage grafts are usually taken from the lower ribs; this rib cartilage requires extensive modeling.

The new cartilage framework obviously must have good skin coverage for the tissue to heal. This is even more important with synthetic materials, so obtaining enough skin may require tissue expansion before surgery; using the fascia from the temple for coverage is an option. A suction drain is used to help the elevated skin attach to the framework. The ear lobule is usually present in cases of microtia. Subsequently, the ear lobule, the tragus (the prominent cartilage in front of the ear), and its canal, are constructed either by repositioning the tissue or using grafts. In the final stage, the entire construct is elevated away from the skull to create a normal prominence of the ear; this step requires skin grafting or a flap of fascia.

In stages when rib cartilages are harvested, several days of hospitalization are usually required; however, the latter stages are usually outpatient procedures, sometimes with overnight observation. The middle ear is usually normal in microtia, but it is important for an otolaryngologist trained in middle ear surgery to evaluate the function of the middle ear and to assist in creating the ear canal when one is not present.

Cryptotia and Constricted Ears: Cup Ears and Lop Ears

Constricted ears are characterized by a band that either limits the diameter of the ear, deepening it enough to create a cuplike appearance, or causing the top portion of the ear to appear to fall forward (lop) over the remaining ear. Infant molding can be effective in the first few months of life but requires constant application as the cartilage stiffens as the estrogen that crossed the placenta leaves the infant's system. Reconstruction is highly variable. The technique needed depends on the severity of the ear anomaly.

Cryptotia refers to ears with the upper portion buried (hidden) beneath the scalp. These ears must be released from the scalp and this band of tissue then reconstructed with grafts or local tissue.

Macrotia: Large Ears and Prominent Ears

Macrotia technically means oversize ears, but prominent ears, which typically are normal size, are often included in this category. Oversize ears can usually be reduced by simple removal of a triangular wedge of cartilage and skin. The ear is then sewn back together with a suture line along the front and back of the ear. Once the stitches are removed and the incision is healed, there should be very little evidence of a scar. Prominent ears are, by far, the most common cosmetic ear complaints. These ears lack a normal antihelical fold, the stiff, inner ridge that curves along the center of the outer ear. This leads the angle between the ear and the skull to widen. This widening may also be caused by an excessive amount of cartilage, referred to as the conchal cartilage, which also pushes the ear away from the scalp.

These can be corrected as an infant with a molding system, as discussed above. Surgery would not be performed until the age of seven to nine typically. The operation to correct protruding ears is known as an otoplasty. The objective of the operation is to reduce the excessive cartilage pushing the ear away from the scalp, to recreate the normal antihelical fold of the ear, and to position the ears so that they lie in a closer, more normal relationship to the scalp. The surgery is performed as an outpatient procedure either in an office-based operating facility or an outpatient operating room. Most children will require general anesthesia, but older children and adults can undergo correction with local anesthesia and sedation. The procedure takes between 1½ and 2½ hours.

The Procedure

The patient is positioned lying flat on the operating-room table, but turning side to side is mandatory. In the most common technique, after sedation and local anesthesia (or general anesthesia in children), a predetermined amount of skin is removed from behind the ear, and the conchal cartilage is identified. If there is excessive ear cartilage, the back surface will be thinned to allow the ear to lie against the side of the head; alternatively, cartilage can be removed. A series of sutures are then placed. One layer of sutures is used to recreate the normal antihelical ear fold, which pulls the helical rim of the ear into a more normal configuration relative to the rest of the ear. A second row of sutures between the conchal cartilage and the mastoid can actually pull the ear back toward the side of the head (see figure 43). Cartilage techniques that do not use sutures include scoring the cartilage so that it slowly unfurls into a more normal position against the scalp or removing a wedge of cartilage to aid in recreating the antihelical fold. Once the ear is repositioned, the incision behind the ear is closed with stitches.

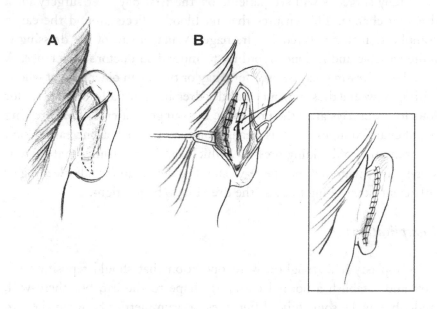

Figure 43. Image of prominent ear incision and surgery

Postoperative Course

After completing the operation, a gauze bandage with a circumferential head dressing will be placed for protection and slight compression. Once the local anesthesia wears off, the ears may have throbbing discomfort or pain that can be moderately severe in some individuals. Usually within twenty-four hours, the pain starts to resolve sufficiently that most patients are quite comfortable. Sleeping with the head elevated may be beneficial, especially if there is a throbbing sensation. The ears will be swollen and bruised in the initial days after surgery. This will have subsided noticeably within a week to ten days postoperatively. The final shape of the ear, however, may not be apparent for several weeks after that. Normal activities can be resumed once the bulky dressing has been removed, but any type of trauma or pulling of the ear forward must be avoided for several more days. Wearing a headband during activities and at night for two to three weeks is helpful. Physical exercise can recommence slowly after the first week to ten days after surgery. Often, absorbable stitches are used in children, but if nonabsorbable sutures are used, they need to be removed one to two weeks after surgery.

Many surgeons will see patients on the first day after surgery for a dressing change. This ensures that no blood collects around the ear, a complication that will require drainage. Management of the dressing is quite variable and is done according to individual doctor's preference. A light head dressing may be used for a day or two in an older patient who is willing to wear a dressing, but a bulkier dressing is usually left in place for four to seven days after the procedure in younger patients. This dressing is not changed unless there is a cause for concern, such as increasing pain or a sensation of building pressure, which can be a warning that there is some problem around the operative site. Problems can include bleeding or sufficient ear swelling to cause the dressing to be too tight.

Complications

Otoplasty is a straightforward operation that should reposition the ears and establish a normal cosmetic shape to the ear, but there will, undoubtedly, be some mild differences or asymmetries between the two sides. This is true of most ears if truly compared, but once ears have been positioned back toward the side of the head, they will no longer be seen at the same time.

As with any operation, there are other potential risks and complications. Fortunately, after otoplasty, they are exceedingly rare but do include bleeding or hematoma, infection, poor cosmesis (appearance), dehiscence (sutures pulling out), and scars. Any collection of blood beneath the incision must be evacuated to prevent infection and warping and/or reabsorption of cartilage. In most instances, the blood can be withdrawn with a needle and syringe. In rare instances, the incision will have to be surgically drained. When the rare infection does occur after otoplasty, it is usually treatable with antibiotics. Any significant infection must be treated promptly and aggressively because it can lead to loss of both cartilage and normal ear contour. Infection is heralded by redness around the incision or ear or drainage of fluid or pus from the wound.

Most patients are delighted with their results, but poor results are, of course, possible. If the rim of the ear is pulled further back toward the head than the position of the newly created ear fold, a "telephone ear" deformity can result where the helix (the normal ear fold) and lobule are much more prominent than the middle of the ear. Similarly, an earlobe or upper pole may not be pulled back to the same degree as the remainder of the ear.

Rarely, an internal suture may break, leading to a partial relapse of the ear projection. This is much more likely in older individuals, as the cartilage is more brittle with age. Scars on and behind the ear generally heal well. But on occasion and more frequently in African Americans, excessive scarring or a true keloid may occur. Either of these would need aggressive management with a cortisone injection and pressure dressings.

Cauliflower Ear: Otohematoma

Cauliflower ear is the term applied to an ear that suffered direct trauma and developed a hematoma but was not seen by the surgeon until long after the hematoma formed (this delayed visit is called late presentation). If the blood is not drained in the acute phase, it leads to deformation, absorption, and thickening of ear cartilage that can lead to a quite deformed ear. Repair requires elevating the skin to expose the cartilage, carving the cartilage to the desired contour, and encouraging reattachment of ear skin with suture and pressure dressings.

Correcting the Large or Small Earlobe

Disproportionate earlobes may occur during child and adolescent growth or develop as an acquired feature from the excess weight of earrings, for example. Operations to enlarge or to reduce the earlobe are relatively straightforward and can be accomplished with local anesthesia in an outpatient setting. Larger lobes are corrected by simply excising a wedge of tissue. The incision is then closed with sutures that are removed about one week after surgery.

Thin earlobes that are either congenital or acquired with advancing age can be corrected with fat injection. Fat is removed with a needle and syringe from an area such as the buttock or lower abdomen. It is then emulsified and reinjected into the earlobe. This is an outpatient procedure that is performed under local anesthesia.

If the earlobe is significantly deficient, it may require augmentation with a skin flap from behind the ear. Although this can also be accomplished under local anesthesia as an outpatient surgery, it is a more sophisticated procedure and will result in a scar behind the ear; this scar should not be very visible. If a large amount of tissue needs to be transferred from behind the ear to the earlobe, a two-stage operation, approximately two weeks apart, may be necessary to preserve blood supply.

Repairing the Torn Earlobe

A partial or complete tear of the earlobe is not uncommon after an ear piercing and is typically caused by a pulling injury on an earring. The torn earlobe can be repaired as an outpatient procedure under local anesthesia, typically in the clinic, in less than thirty minutes. After cleaning the ear and introducing the local anesthetic, the tear in the earlobe is removed, and reconstruction commences either in a straight line or in a planned pattern to optimize the appearance and scar position. The earlobe is then reconstructed with a row of stitches in the skin in front of and behind the ear. Sutures are removed after one week, and the ear can be safely repierced a month or so later if a small hole was not intentionally left at the time of repair. These repairs are more complicated with larger defects, as is often seen with ear gauges, which stretch out the earlobe, and a simple repair would lead to a long, thin earlobe. Tissue rearrangement is necessary to optimize these results and are case dependent.

Such repairs are minor procedures with little postoperative discomfort. Complications are rare but can include bleeding, infection, and cyst formation. Infection is characterized by swelling, redness, and discomfort and will usually respond to oral antibiotics. If a lump in the suture line develops after repair, it is most commonly caused by a piece of retained skin in the scar line, which creates a cyst. This cyst will not resolve and needs to be surgically removed under local anesthesia.

THE BREAST

To understand the human breast, we must remember that humans are mammals. In addition to being warm-blooded, breathing oxygen, and having hair or fur, mammals have milk-producing breasts with which females feed their young. For this reason, the breast is known as the mammary gland: *mammal* and *mammary* are closely related words. In men, the mammary gland does not produce milk. In adolescent girls and women, it responds to the hormones secreted from the ovary and from the pituitary gland in the brain, changing its functions with various events in life: puberty, pregnancy, lactation (breast-feeding), and menopause.

The circular, globular, symmetrical shape of the female breasts provides a silhouette that represents a part of sensuous beauty that is as important in humans as is the breasts' ability to produce milk. This reality causes many women to seek reconstructive help to attain perfection in size and contour.

Breast Development

Before birth, a ridge develops on each side of an embryo's body. This ridge extends from the armpit (the axilla) to the groin; as the embryo develops, this ridge typically disappears except for a small area on each side of the chest, from which the future breasts develop. The breast tissue remains quiescent throughout childhood, beginning to develop at puberty, when the ovaries begin secreting estrogen and progesterone. Both males and females may develop firm lumps beneath the nipples before puberty. This condition probably results from normal hormonal stimulation of the breast tissue. It is usually complete in one to two years.

Genetics, diet, and hormones influence the size of a normal, healthy woman's breasts. Layers of tough, soft tissues called fascia surround the adult mammary gland. A space behind the breast permits the breast—and the fascia layers that hold it—to move more freely on the chest wall. The layers of fascia enveloping the breast are somewhat loose, and this looseness increases with age and will predispose the breast to sagging. These changes are often exacerbated after pregnancy, as the milk-producing breast may more than double in weight. The layers of fascia are unable to reconform to their state before pregnancy, leading them to sag when lactation ends.

Breast Anatomy

The developed female breast is shaped like a cone that extends vertically between the second and eighth ribs and across the front from the sternum (breastbone) to an imaginary line below the armpit (this line is called the anterior axillary line). A portion of the breast tissue extends into the armpit and is referred to as the Tail of Spence, named for Dr. James Spence, who first defined it. The breast is made of glands and ducts, which are divided into lobes (or sections). These lobes are surrounded by connective and fatty tissues. The skin overlying the breast is thin and contains sweat glands, oil-secreting glands, and hair follicles. The dark, wrinkled skin containing the nipple is called the areola. Ducts inside the breast drain from the breast glands to the nipple, carrying milk during lactation.

The breast has many more nerves than most parts of the body, and the majority of nerves come from the spaces between the ribs. The most important one is the nerve to the nipple-areola complex, which originates on the side of the chest between the fourth and fifth ribs. It passes between the breasts and underlying muscle and then continues upward into the breast. Inside the breast, it finally divides to provide sensation to the nipple-areola complex.

Potential Breast Abnormalities

There are a number of potential abnormalities in breast development:

1. Abnormality of size
   a. Absence of breast development (amastia)
   b. Small or undeveloped breasts (hypomastia)
   c. Heavy, pendulous breasts (macromastia)
2. Abnormalities of shape: congenital and acquired
3. Excessive male breast tissue (gynecomastia)
4. Extra tissue
   a. Breast tissue located outside the main breasts
   b. Nipples numbering more than two (polythelia)
5. Loss of breast due to trauma, breast cancer, etc.
6. Changes that may occur as a consequence of pregnancy, nursing, and aging

UNDESIRED BREASTS

Gynecomastia (Breasts on a Man)

Men have breasts but with minimal glandular tissue present. Gynecomastia refers to the development of female-quantity breast glands in the male patient. Most cases begin during puberty. No one knows why certain adolescent males develop breast tissue, but it is probably caused by having either higher levels of hormones in the blood or an increased sensitivity of normal breast tissue to typical levels of circulating hormones, especially the female hormone called estrogen. Alternatively, it may be due to either decreased levels of male hormones (such as testosterone) or insensitivity to these hormones.

Gynecomastia is more common than one might think, affecting up to 40% of young men at some point during their adolescence. Either one or both breasts may be affected. Most cases of gynecomastia will resolve within two to three years, not becoming sufficiently problematic to require a young man to seek medical attention. If a large amount of breast tissue develops or a moderate amount fails to disappear, gynecomastia can be a source of considerable embarrassment to young men. Older men develop some amount of gynecomastia because less testosterone is made and more testosterone (a male hormone) converts to estrogen (a female hormone) in the body.

Certain medications and drugs, such as marijuana and anabolic steroids, can cause gynecomastia. Further, several medical conditions can stimulate the development of breast tissue in males, including liver disease; alcoholism; kidney failure; abnormalities of the adrenal glands; tumors of the testes, lung, adrenal glands, or pituitary gland. Gynecomastia can also result from genetic errors in a person's chromosomes, especially Klinefelter's syndrome, which also carries with it a high risk for breast cancer.

The Consultation and Plan

If one seeks surgery to correct gynecomastia, the surgeon must take a careful medical and social history and perform a thorough physical exam, including an exam of the breasts, the abdominal organs, and the testes. Because hormones and genetic factors can cause gynecomastia, the plastic surgeon may need to refer a patient to an endocrinologist for either (1) blood and urine studies that would show elevated hormone levels or (2) genetic studies that would show the count and other details of the patient's chromosomes. An abnormal testicular exam will prompt the surgeon to order an ultrasound of the testes. The surgeon may wish to obtain a mammogram to rule out a breast tumor, which, though unlikely, can occur in men, especially with asymmetric breast development.

Even though these medical conditions are possible causes of gynecomastia, the overwhelming majority of cases have no known cause and no associated medical problems. In these cases, treatment will focus only on surgically correcting the gynecomastia.

It is important to examine the breasts to determine the amount of excess skin and which component of the enlarged tissues is fat and which is true breast tissue. Breast tissue is firm or hard, while fat feels soft. Individuals whose larger breasts are made mainly of fatty tissue can be treated with liposuction. By using liposuction that is assisted by energy (ultrasound or laser), the surgeon has greater ability to break loose and remove dense fat and breast tissue. In addition, energy-assisted liposuction is thought to improve the cosmetic result because it appears to tighten the skin by applying heat that causes the skin's collagen to shrink.

If there is hard breast tissue, a large breast plate, or noticeably excessive skin, these will typically need to be removed surgically despite energy-assisted liposuction. In most cases, the operation can be done through an incision that is limited to—and hidden in—the lower half of the areola, which is the dark skin that surrounds the nipple. It is preferable not to remove skin. If there is a large, hanging breast with a lot of extra skin, skin may have to be removed. This will create scars on the breast skin outside the areola, similar to a breast lift.

The Procedure

The operation is usually performed on an outpatient basis. Depending on the size of the breasts and surgeon's preference, it often can be done with sedation and local anesthesia. Large corrections may require general anesthesia. In some instances, a one-night admission to the hospital may be necessary.

If correction is being done with liposuction only (with or without assistance from laser or ultrasound), scars are usually limited to small incisions in the areola or under the armpit. The excess fat and extra breast tissue will be pretreated and then liposuctioned. A dressing of gauze and compression bandages or garments will be applied and maintained for a couple weeks for compression.

If surgical removal of breast tissue or excess skin is necessary, larger incisions will be made (1) through the areola; (2) around the nipple; or (3) on the breast tissue, either at the lower breast or with scars similar to those seen in procedures for a breast lift (mastopexy) or a breast reduction These may include a vertical incision from the nipple to the fold below the breast; sometimes, an incision with a subsequent scar along the lower breast fold itself is needed.

On occasion, the extra breast or fatty tissue will be removed while leaving excess skin, in hopes that the skin will resolve, or retract to a smaller size. If the skin does not redrape itself appropriately, there will be loose, excess skin overlying the area where the breast tissue previously existed, and a second operation to remove the excess skin will be necessary. This procedure can usually be performed in the clinic under local anesthesia. This approach is sometimes advantageous in that fewer scars may result in the end. This is a fact that the surgeon and patient must carefully discuss before surgery is undertaken.

Recovery

The chest will be swollen and bruised for several days to weeks. Depending on the amount of tissue and excess skin removed, wearing a compression bandage will be necessary for one to six weeks. Sutures are removed between one and two weeks after surgery. Recuperation is rapid in most cases. There may be some pain and discomfort in the initial days, requiring prescription medication. The pain will resolve quickly, and the patient should be able to return to work or light activities within several days. With larger removals of tissue and/or skin, it may be seven to ten days before returning to work and light activities is recommended. After removal of the sutures, a patient may return to activity quite quickly, but strenuous activity should be avoided for about three weeks. If significant surgical removal of breast tissue and/or skin is performed, the surgeon may need to use drainage tubes to remove blood and fluids that collect under the incision. The drainage tube will be removed as soon as the drainage stops, usually between one and five days after surgery.

Any patient with realistic expectations should be very satisfied with the results of surgery. In most instances, patients are pleased with the correction and possess a flat, normal-appearing chest with scars, as mentioned. Scars in the areola or under the armpit usually settle down nicely and are difficult to see. Nevertheless, if larger areas of skin must be removed, the resulting scars in the chest skin can be quite noticeable. They will remain red for at least three months, and then the redness will slowly fade. The scars will take about a year to settle into their final appearance.

Complications

As with any operation, gynecomastia surgery has potential risks and complications. They are infrequent but include bleeding, nipple retraction, nipple loss (or nipple death), reduced nipple sensation, and breast asymmetry. Men should also recognize that breast cancer may be found during gynecomastia surgery.

Active bleeding can be a complication that would require a second operation to stop the bleeding and to drain any accumulation of blood; this is called a hematoma.

Removing the breast plate and breast tissue may lead to nipple retraction, which means that the nipple does not adequately project from the chest. This may be treated with an implantation or injection of fat. Another possible complication involving the nipple is nipple loss, but complete or partial nipple death is a very rare complication because the operation is designed to maintain adequate blood supply to the nipple. Yet, if the nipple and surrounding areola die because of an insufficient blood supply, they would require removal; this problem is then treated with dressing changes to aid healing. The nipple could be reconstructed at a later date, but nipple reconstructions have limited sensation.

Nipple sensation can be reduced after gynecomastia surgery, but it will usually return to normal in several weeks or months. In rare instances, sensation may remain reduced or absent.

Corrected breasts may not be symmetrical. The surgeon's goal is to correct the breasts so that they are equal in appearance, but any difference in size, shape, or nipple position may need correction in a second operation.

Even in men, breast cancer does occur. Therefore, all removed tissue may be sent for examination by a pathologist. Rarely, this examination will reveal unexpected breast cancer. Any cancer diagnosis will require additional evaluation and treatment.

Polymastia (Extra Breasts)

Having an extra breast, called polymastia, exists in nearly 1% of the population, and the extra breast may or may not have a nipple. If an extra breast has no nipple, it is difficult to tell whether it is truly an extra breast or actually accessory (extra) breast tissue of one of the two normal breasts. Breast tissue can develop before birth anywhere along the fetal mammary ridge (milk line), which extends from the armpit to the lower abdomen and even beyond, into the groin.

Most frequently, extra breasts grow in the armpit. Some individuals have a soft mound of extra breast tissue either overhanging the bra or bathing-suit strap or lying below the normal breast in the lower part of the chest. In many patients, the excess is fat tissue; however, in some, it is made up of extra breast glands and other essential structures of the breast. These deposits of breast tissue may be uncomfortable because they interfere with clothing, and they may be unattractive. They can also develop the same benign and malignant breast diseases that normal breast tissue can.

Small deposits of extra breast tissue can be removed with liposuction, but larger areas and the excess skin that overlies them may need to be surgically removed. Scars are usually hidden in the armpit or in the fold where the lower portion of the normal breast (that the patient will keep) curves back to meet the chest wall.

When an extra breast has a nipple, both skin and nipple must be removed. A small extra breast can be removed under local anesthesia. Removing a larger extra breast may require sedation or general anesthesia. Stitches are removed within eight to fourteen days. There may be pain after surgery that requires prescription pain medication for several days. Patients may return to normal activities within seven to ten days and to strenuous activities within three weeks.

Polythelia (Extra Nipples)

Accessory nipples can also occur anywhere along the milk line (see above); however, the majority of extra nipples are seen below the level of the normal nipple. The accessory nipples may exist alone or may be surrounded by the dark skin of the areola. They may also overlie accessory breast tissue. Extra nipples are a common finding, occurring in 0.2% to 2.5% of the population (that is, two to twenty-five persons per thousand). They occur in both sexes, but interestingly, they are seen more commonly in males. In half of patients with polythelia, extra nipples are found on both sides of the body.

An accessory nipple can be removed, but doing so will leave a small scar at the site of removal. Removal is a simple office procedure that can be done under local anesthesia. Stitches are removed within eight to fourteen days, and regular activity may be resumed immediately after the procedure.

BREAST REDUCTION

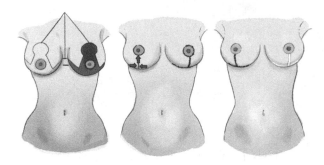

Figure 44

There are no known causes behind developing excessively large breasts (macromastia), but current science suggests that greater sensitivity of breast cells to normal levels of estrogen may be responsible. Macromastia may also occur because of genetic predisposition or significant weight gain.

Teenagers may develop very large breasts soon after the onset of menstruation. This is known as virginal hypertrophy. Young teenagers with very large breasts who suffer from significant psychological trauma are candidates for breast-reduction surgery, which is also called reduction mammoplasty. In some instances, it is preferable to wait until breasts are fully developed before operating. The breast tissue will not regrow in most instances, but young teenagers and their parents must know that as the teen continues to develop, the breasts may again enlarge, requiring repeat breast-reduction surgery.

Heavy, pendulous breasts can cause many problems. The heavy weight often leads to progressive pain in the neck and upper back because of muscle tightness and spasms. The weight of the breasts on bra straps may cause uncomfortable or even painful indentations and grooves on the shoulders. Some women experience episodes of numbness and tingling. Furthermore, the sagging breasts lie against the lower chest and upper abdomen, trapping sweat and causing irritation and rashes known as intertrigo. Finally, large breasts that are disproportional to the rest of the body can be a source of considerable embarrassment, especially for teenagers and younger women. Women experiencing any of these problems may be candidates for breast reduction.

The Consultation

It is important to have an idea of the planned size of the breasts. Breast size will need to be coordinated with overall body size and shape. Breast reduction is designed to remove extra skin, fat, and breast tissue while also returning the pendulous breasts to a more normal contour and position on the chest wall. Large areolas can also be reduced to a more aesthetically pleasing size. Breast reduction is not considered an elective cosmetic operation, per se, but rather a reconstructive operation that results in a healthier, more comfortable quality of life if enough tissue is removed. Although the surgery may be considered to be medically necessary, it is carried out in such a way as to provide the most aesthetic breasts possible. In some cases, it is necessary to perform liposuction of the lateral chest roll leading up to the breasts. This is not actually breast tissue but can be important from a cosmetic perspective. This frequently involves out-of-pocket expense as it is not medically necessary in many cases.

At the initial consultation, the surgeon will take a detailed medical history, including any history of breast cancer on the patient's mother side of the family. All patients over forty years of age will need to have a current mammogram before undergoing reduction mammoplasty. To prove that the procedure is medically necessary, the surgeon will gather information required by insurance companies: measurements and photographs, in addition to a detailed history of complaints, efforts that have been made to alleviate complaints, and an estimate of the amount of tissue the surgeon believes will need to be removed. The breasts will be measured with special attention to the location of the nipple relative to the collarbone and the lower breast fold.

The Options

It is important to discuss where the surgical scars will be and what the patient should expect after surgery. Although an outstanding operation may remedy all previous concerns and provide nicely positioned, attractive breasts, the operation will nevertheless result in breast scars. In order to remove the extra skin and breast tissue and to recreate a cone-shaped breast, scars may extend around the areola and from the areola down along the lower portion of the breasts to the inframammary fold, where they may meet a third scar extending across the full width of the inframammary fold for lower and larger breasts. The amount of scarring is highly variable—it depends on breast characteristics, the skin, a patient's genetics, healing events, and the surgical technique used. The scars are usually well hidden beneath a bra or even a bathing suit or low-cut dress but are never invisible. Because complaints and symptoms from before surgery are typically improved, the scars are usually extremely well tolerated.

A number of operative procedures can be used to reduce the size of the breast. The most common operation uses a keyhole-shaped incision in which the nipple and areola are left attached to breast tissue and blood vessels from the lower base of the breast. The nipple is then brought up to its new position on the chest; this operation, which uses an inferior blood supply, is known as the inferior pedicle technique. Extra skin, fat, and breast tissue are removed, and extra fat at the side of the breast and chest extending upward, toward the armpit, can be removed by liposuction. The incisions are closed, and the suture line is usually covered with Steri-Strips or butterfly tapes. This technique's major advantages are that it is very dependable, provides immediate results during surgery that can easily be fine-tuned, and has the smallest effects on subsequent breast function (i.e., sensation, breast-feeding, etc.). The major disadvantage is the amount of scarring it causes.

The most common alternative techniques are geared toward scar reduction. These are usually superior or superomedial pedicle techniques, aimed at eliminating or reducing the breast scar underneath: collectively referred to as vertical reduction mammoplasty. The blood supply for breast tissue moved in these techniques is from the upper chest and breast. The major advantages are increased projection of the nipple and the possibility of eliminating—or at least shortening—the scar at the base of the breast. This technique has a less satisfying immediate result, however, as the closure requires leaving bunched-up tissue where the vertical incision is closed. Over time, this tissue loosens and stretches, usually with better projection, but this process may take one to three months to occur and may not completely smooth out.

Some patients may find it difficult to wait for the uncertainty and delay of seeing the final result of vertical reduction mammoplasty. Also, the inability to perfectly predict the final result impairs the surgeon's ability to fine-tune final appearance on the operating table. Thus, a second, minor, revision surgery is more frequently necessary with these procedures. It can be difficult to apply to larger breast reductions. In short, these reduced-scar techniques are best applied to moderate macromastia, but expert surgeons can use and modify them for severe macromastia.

If patients have extremely large breasts (gigantomastia), the nipples and areolas may not survive being moved to a higher position on the breast because the blood vessels moved with them may not supply adequate blood supply for the large amount of tissue. If the surgeon suspects that moving the nipple and areola may cause these structures to die or identifies this during or soon after surgery, a reduction mammoplasty that grafts the nipple and areola to a new location may be advised. This technique is very similar to the previously described operation, except that the nipple and areola are temporarily removed from the breasts. At the end of the operation, they are placed in their new locations as a skin graft. The graft transfer is usually successful, although there is always the risk of loss, should the nipple and areola die. Some patients will experience abnormal pigmentation (color) in the grafted nipple and areola. This is most frequently noted in darker-skinned patients. Other disadvantages include the likely loss of sensation, nipple projection, and the ability to breast-feed a future child.

The Procedure

Breast reduction surgery usually involves minimal blood loss, but because this is elective, some surgeons may have certain high-risk patients donate a unit of their own blood one to three weeks before surgery.

Immediately before surgery, the breasts will be marked with the patient sitting or standing in an upright position—as it can be very difficult to establish symmetry once the patient is lying on her back if the two sides were not previously marked. The new nipple position will be marked at or just above the inframammary fold. Markings for the incision will then be planned. During the surgery, the nipples are moved, the excess skin and breast tissue are removed, and any necessary liposuction is completed. The breasts are then closed, frequently with a drain to evacuate blood and fluid from the surgical site.

Recovery

The breasts will be tender and swollen after the operation, with breast- and chest-wall discomfort, although pain is not necessarily severe. Any pain will usually subside after several days and can be controlled with prescribed medications. Even so, it is not unusual for patients to experience episodes of discomfort or even shooting pains in the initial months after the operation, as nerve endings regenerate.

The breasts are bandaged with gauze dressings after surgery. The bandages may be changed after several days; the breasts will then be dressed with light gauze and a bra or compression garment. The swelling and bruising will subside over several weeks. If drains are placed, they will typically be removed between one and seven days after the operation, when drainage has nearly stopped. Stitches are removed between ten days and three weeks.

Physical activity should be very limited for the first seven to ten days after the surgery, and it will be three weeks before more normal activities can be resumed. Strenuous physical activity and exercise should be avoided for six weeks. It will take about three months for the breasts to settle and achieve their new appearance, especially with the vertical reduction techniques.

Subtle changes will continue for at least six to twelve months after surgery, as the breasts continue to soften and drop. There may be some relapse of sagging. The scars will become redder and wider in the initial months after surgery, and then fade and flatten for up to eighteen months. If the scars fail to do so, they may need cortisone injections, scar cream, and/or compression with silicone, which surgeons have found to reduce scarring.

It is important to obtain a baseline mammogram one year after breast-reduction surgery because the procedure changes the breast's appearance in images.

Complications

Bleeding and Infection

Although rare, bleeding and collections of blood, called hematomas, are complications that can require a patient to undergo reoperation under anesthesia to evacuate old blood and control bleeding.

Mild skin infections, though infrequent, can often be controlled with oral antibiotics. Rarely, a deeper infection can occur underneath the breast tissue, and the incision will have to be surgically opened and the area drained.

Tissue Loss

Cigarette smokers are more likely than nonsmokers to experience the complications of nipple loss, skin loss, death of fatty tissue (fat necrosis), and delayed healing of incisions, but it can occur in anyone, and the risks increase with vascular diseases such as hypertension or arterial disease as skin survival is dependent on blood supply.

If skin loss does occur, it is usually confined to a small area where the vertical scar and the scar in the inframammary fold meet, below the breast. This complication can usually be treated with topical antibiotics and minor incision care. However, skin loss across larger areas can occur, which again can usually be managed by removing damaged or infected tissue from the affected area and providing incision care. Only rarely may additional surgery or prolonged incision care be necessary.

Although it is extremely rare, nipple loss is the most feared complication of breast reduction. Because the nipple and areola have a reduced blood supply after surgery, blood flow may be inadequate to nourish them once incisions are made. This can result in total nipple and areola loss. Should this happen, additional operations are required to get the incisions clean and closed. The nipple can then be reconstructed later (see details on nipple reconstruction).

Patients undergoing breast reductions can develop fat necrosis—areas that are either firm or tender and hard—due to inadequate blood supply to small areas of fat underneath the skin. In most instances, these areas will soften and resolve with time. They may, however, calcify and appear on mammograms; this is one reason for the required baseline mammogram one year after breast reduction, mentioned above. If fat necrosis becomes exposed, it complicates the healing process and may require removal of devitalized tissue and dressing changes.

Concerns during Healing

The typical and more immediate complications of breast reduction are scarring, breast asymmetry, and nipple sensation.

Prominent scarring is the most common cause of patient dissatisfaction. Patients need to know and agree with the incisions and subsequent scars necessary to achieve the desired result before they undergo surgery. Patients with a history of poor scarring should treat scars prophylactically with scar cream or silicone sheeting. Laser therapy can be beneficial as well.

Breast asymmetry may result from preoperative asymmetry or operative changes. It is important to note differences in breast shape and size before surgery and plan accordingly, but perfect symmetry is very rarely achieved. Unacceptable asymmetry may require additional corrective surgery if desired.

It is not uncommon after breast reduction to have a period of decreased sensitivity in the nipples. In most instances, normal sensation will return. There is always the possibility, however, of permanent numbness or altered sensation in the nipple, especially with areola- and nipple-grafting techniques. Some patients will complain of increased sensitivity in the nipple area during the recovery process and for several weeks after the operation. This usually normalizes.

A rare complication would be an unexpected diagnosis of breast cancer. If this occurs, a mastectomy is frequently recommended because breast-reduction tissue comes from many different parts of the breast and it can be hard to determine where an unexpected malignancy came from.

BREAST LIFT (MASTOPEXY)

Mastopexy (Breast-Lift Surgery)

Sagging of the breasts is referred to as breast ptosis. Breast-lift surgery, or mastopexy, is an operation designed to raise the sagging breasts to a more normal position on the chest. As women age—especially after pregnancy and nursing—the breast's skin will loosen and will sag more and more and become less shapely. Breast ptosis is classified by the position of the nipple and areola relative to the inframammary fold, where the lower portion of the breast and the chest meet, as shown in the box, below.

Mild sagging (1st-degree ptosis): The nipple is at the level of the inframammary fold.

Moderate sagging (2nd-degree ptosis): The nipple has fallen just below the inframammary fold but remains above the most projected portion of the breast.

Severe sagging (3rd-degree ptosis): The nipple has fallen well below the fold and is pointing downward.

"False" sagging (Pseudoptosis): The nipple is appropriately positioned, but the lower breast bottoms out; or the nipple lies at the level of the inframammary fold, but the lower portions of the breasts have descended well below the inframammary fold.

The Options

At the initial consultations with a plastic surgeon, a patient must discuss her concerns relating to her breasts' size, shape, and position. After pregnancies and breast-feeding, the breasts may develop deflation hypomastia. After lactation, a breast can both sag and lose volume in the upper portion. Women experiencing this phenomenon generally feel that their breasts both sag and are smaller than desired. Push-up bras will often camouflage this problem while women are clothed, but correction will require surgery. In the case of mild ptosis and deflation hypomastias, a breast implant alone may correct the deformity. The advantages of this are the resulting minimal scar necessary to place an implant and improve upper-breast fullness. Patients must be willing to undergo placement of a breast implant. If a significant lift is necessary, a formal mastopexy will be required.

Mastopexy will lift the breasts to a more ideal location on the chest, but it is important to realize that over time, the breasts will sag again. Smaller breasts will take longer to sag again than larger, heavier breasts or breasts with loose fascia or skin. If a woman who underwent mastopexy were to have another child or have another reason for significant weight fluctuations, it is quite likely that the breasts would sag to some extent, although typically less. Thus, it is usually recommended to complete all pregnancies before undergoing mastopexy. If a woman does bear a child after mastopexy, breast-feeding should not be impaired because many ducts are not disrupted. Many women find breast-feeding after a lift easier. However, scars may make breast-feeding more difficult or painful.

For a patient's safety, the surgeon will examine the breasts to make sure there are no lumps. A mammogram before any surgery is done is recommended for women over forty and for a patient with a strong maternal family history of breast cancer.

The biggest drawback to any breast-lift operation is the amount of scarring on the breasts. To correct a sagging breast, excess skin must be removed; this necessarily results in a scar. The operations are designed so that any scars are hidden beneath a modest bathing suit or bra, and the scars typically do very well. The type of surgery and amount of scarring will depend on the degree of sagging. Moderate ptosis can be corrected by excising skin in a doughnut fashion around the areola; the scar is limited to the circumference of the areola. More skin can be removed, between the six-o'clock position of the areola and the inframammary fold; this results in a tennis-racket-shaped scar. Often, however, even more skin needs to be removed; in this case, the resulting scar is shaped like an anchor, extending around the circumference of the areola, vertically down the lower portion of the breast and then horizontally along the inframammary fold, similar to a breast lift. Regardless of the approach, all operations are designed to move the nipple and areola to a higher position and to create a firmer, shapely breast.

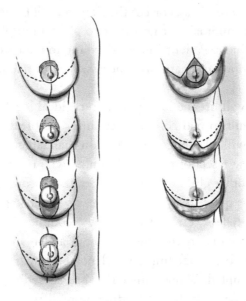

Figure 45: Various Types of breast lift procedures

The Procedure

The operation will usually take from $1^1/_2$ to 3 hours. The procedure is performed either under general anesthesia with the patient asleep or with heavy sedation and local anesthesia to numb the breasts. The operation is typically carried out on an outpatient basis or with overnight observation.

Incisions and the new nipple position are marked on the skin while the patient is sitting or standing up, before the operation begins. After the surgery begins, these marked incisions are made, the extra skin is removed, the breasts are repositioned, and the wounds are closed with stitches. Steri-Strips (narrow surgical tapes) are usually placed over the suture line. Gauze bandages are held in place with a surgical bra or a bandage wrapped around the body.

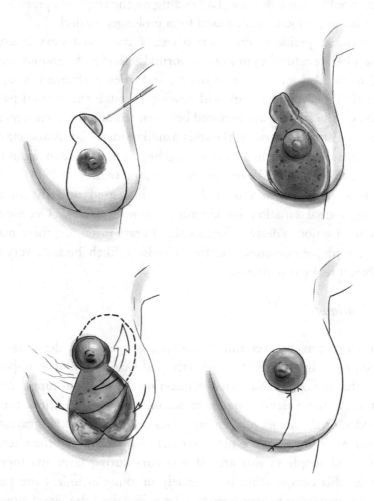

Figure 46: Sequence of events in superomedial pedicle mastopexy

Recovery

For the first few days, the breasts will be tender, bruised, swollen, and covered with a gauze bandage. Pain will resolve in several days and can be easily treated with prescribed medication. The swelling and tenderness will begin to subside after several days, but it will take three to four weeks to fully resolve. It can take up to three months for the final result to be apparent, although subtle changes will continue for up to a year largely characterized by some descent. Depending on the surgeon's preference, a support bra or garment may be used for a prolonged period.

A recovery period of one to two weeks after mastopexy is usually necessary before returning to work or normal activities. Strenuous activity should be avoided for four to six weeks, and when performed, a support bra should be used. The scars will develop through the normal pattern of healing. The stitches are removed between ten and fourteen days after surgery, and after this is done, the scars usually widen slightly and may itch and become red. The redness and itching begins to subside in about three months, and the scars will continue to fade for a year.

Nipple sensation may be reduced or increased initially. In most instances, normal sensation should return after several weeks. Occasionally, return of sensation is delayed for months. In rare instances, there may be permanent nipple numbness, yet this is most unlikely because very little to no breast tissue is removed.

Complications

Ptosis may recur over time because mastopexy is a delaying tactic intended to fight the effects of gravity and skin laxity. It is important to note that removing skin places tension on the scar and nipple-areolar complex. As these tissues stretch to accommodate the tension, the scar may widen or the areola may enlarge. Besides infection, the gravest risk of mastopexy is death of the nipple-areolar complex due to the alteration of the blood supply to this area that occurs during large mastopexies. However, this complication is extremely uncommon unless the patient has had previous breast surgeries that have impaired the blood supply to the nipple and the areola. The other complications are all similar to breast reduction.

BREAST AUGMENTATION

Breast Augmentation

Breast augmentation, or augmentation mammoplasty, is a surgical technique to increase breast size. There is no "normal" breast size or shape for any given woman, but each woman has her own ideal. If she desires a larger breast, she may wish to undergo breast augmentation. Many women are satisfied with their breast size and shape until a structural change has taken place after pregnancy and breast-feeding, causing deflation and sagging, mainly of the upper portion of the breast. Ideally, the woman choosing augmentation surgery should have realistic expectations in anticipating improved body shape and appearance. Those hoping for more dramatic life changes may be disappointed.

The Consultation

In the consultations before the operation, it is important that the patient discuss her desires and concerns very carefully with her plastic surgeon. The patient should be involved in the decision as to where the incision for placement of the breast implant is to be made. She needs to understand the implant's placement and depth relative to the breast, muscle, and chest wall.

The patient must thoroughly discuss the breast size she would like to have so that the surgeon will understand her expectations. This is often more difficult to determine than one may expect. It is important to note that breast cup sizes vary widely by brassiere manufacturer. The patient may use external sizers or bags filled with water to estimate the desired size, but this technique has limited precision. In selecting a breast size, the woman's natural body size and shape must be considered, as well as the distortions that can occur from too large an implant and the frustrations that can result from too small an implant. Photographs of a patient's goals from popular media or catalogs can be helpful. Complicated morphing software can use 3-D imaging to assist in picking a size but can still be less than perfect. The most important ingredient is communication from the patient to the physician and a joint decision between the two.

The patient also needs to discuss any concerns she has related to her breast and nipple position, including any associated asymmetry or sagging of the breasts. In certain instances, the implant alone can correct sagging, but additional surgery (i.e., breast lift or mastopexy) may be required, either simultaneously or in a delayed fashion for more symmetry. All breasts are asymmetric and still will be after augmentation, but they are typically more similar after augmentation than before.

Breast health is also important. The surgeon will examine the breasts to make certain there are no lumps or other problems. If the patient has a family history of breast cancer on the mother's side, or if she is forty years old or older, a mammogram may be ordered before surgery.

The Options

Type of Implant

Breast augmentation is accomplished by placing a silicone shell filled with normal saline (salt water) or silicone gel into the breast. For many years in the United States, gel-filled implants were not approved by the United States Food and Drug Administration (FDA) for cosmetic breast augmentation. This started with the highly publicized controversy regarding the long-term health consequences of using silicone gel implants in the 1980s. During this time, gel-filled implants remained available for breast reconstruction after mastectomy, for reconstruction of congenital deformities, and for women who had a complication with previously inserted silicone implants (but only as part of an FDA study). Silicone gel implants were also available in most countries outside the United States.

The findings of all research studies to date have failed to demonstrate a relationship between silicone gel and systemic (body-wide) illness, and in 2006, silicone gel implants were again approved for cosmetic breast surgery. These implants are far more technologically advanced than the early models were, and the slow silicone leak that was felt to be responsible for most of the local problems with silicone implants is either very slight or does not occur. Another style of implants that has been developed is the cohesive gel implant, which maintains a solid form even without the solid external shell. These implants have a stabilized and more dense form.

There are also options for breast-implant shape. The most commonly used implants are round, which become shaped because of the influence of gravity. The anatomic implants attempt to replicate the breast shape with a teardrop pattern, larger at the bottom than at the top. The rare but potential disadvantage of using the anatomic implant is that obvious deformities may occur if the implant becomes rotated or are otherwise malpositioned. Shaped implants are textured, as discussed below, so as to help minimize these problems, but due to the friction of the texture, a malpositioned implant is difficult to correct without a surgical procedure either in the office or in the OR.

The implants available in the United States have either a smooth or textured silicone wall. Results in augmentation mammoplasty have been very good with either type. Proponents of the textured implants believe that the complication of soft-tissue hardening (capsular contracture) around the breast implants occurs less often with these. Textured implants also tend to move less over time, important with large implants, combination breast lift with implant surgeries, and with shaped (i.e., teardrop-shaped implants) where a turn of the implant could lead to distortion. Proponents of the smooth-walled implants believe that the resulting contour and appearance of the breasts are smoother and less rippled and that the movement of the smooth implant is more natural.

Implants also come in different profiles, meaning the amount of projection. Higher-profile implants have a narrower base, giving the breasts increased projection. These are particularly useful in patients with thin, narrow chests. Higher-profile implants also allow for a larger implant to fit a given chest without being too wide, which can lead to the breasts being too close (symmastia) or hanging off the side of the chest. Some of this is based on the patient's preference.

The aesthetic difference between silicone and saline is quite subjective and a frequent victim of bias. However, it is universally felt that gel implants maintain a softer, more natural feel than saline implants do, especially in patients with less of their own breast tissue. Saline implants are also more prone to rippling, being round in the upper chest and being more firm. The leak rate is actually higher in saline implants due to the extra valve used to fill the implant (see below).

Silicone implants do require larger incisions (about 5 cm for gel and 6 cm for cohesives) than their saline counterparts (about 3 cm), which are implanted empty and then filled. This also adds some adjustability to saline implants.

Options for Incisions

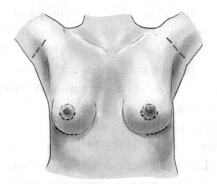

Figure 47: Authors Common Incisions for Breast Augmentation

The implant may be inserted by four different incisions or approaches:

The periareolar incision is made around a portion (up to half) of the circumference of the areola, keeping the incision off the adjacent breast skin. Theoretically, this incision has a higher risk of altered nipple sensation and impairment of breast-feeding, but most research studies have failed to show a significant difference in rates of either of these. In certain breasts, this approach provides both adequate space for the surgeon to work and a nearly imperceptible scar. The areola needs to be large enough to accommodate the length of scar necessary to insert a silicone implant. This technique may be beneficial when there is a need to reduce the size of the nipple-areola complex or to perform a mastopexy (breast lift) during the same procedure. A slightly higher risk of capsular contracture has been demonstrated likely due to contamination from some of the bacteria in the breast ducts.

The inframammary incision is made in the breast's lower aspect, just above the inframammary fold, where the lower breast meets the chest. Despite concerns about this scar's visibility, it is usually well hidden below the breast in the inframammary fold. This approach provides the best access for the surgeon to work, especially in cases that require supplemental breast procedures, such as managing cases of significant asymmetry of breast size or position. It also violates the least amount of breast tissue and nipple blood supply.

The transaxillary incision is made in the armpit, keeping scars off the breasts. The surgeon's access to the breast and ability to release tight muscle bands, correct asymmetry, and revise the position of the inframammary fold are limited with this technique. These issues are improved when an endoscope is used. Patients must be aware that if complications like severe bleeding or poor visibility occur with this technique, a second incision may need to be made on the breast to complete the surgery. While this approach avoids a scar on the breast, it does leave a scar in the axilla. It is usually well hidden but may be visible in a tank top or bathing suit when the arms are raised. A higher rate of capsular contracture and revisional surgery have been seen with this technique by the authors.

Implants may be placed via the abdominal area. In the transumbilical approach, an incision is made in the belly button. A tube is then used to pass a saline implant from the navel to the breast. The surgeon must use an endoscope. As with the transaxillary approach, discussed above, the same risk of a second incision on the breast being made for urgent problems exists. This approach voids the warranty of the implant as the implant is much more likely to be damaged during the tunneled placement. Also, asymmetric results are more common due to decreased exposure. An additional option is to place the implants at the time of an abdominoplasty through the elevated abdominal flap prior to closure.

Depth of Implant Placement

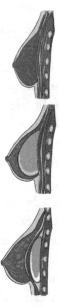

Figure 48: Authors Common Placement Options for Breast Implant Depth

Surgeons can insert implants at different depths. The implants may be placed beneath the breasts either (1) above the pectoralis major muscle and fascia (submammary placement), just above the pectoralis muscle but below the fascia (subfascial), or (2) below the pectoralis major muscle, above the rib cage (submuscular placement), or a combination approach (dual plane). Silicone implants can be placed in any location with aesthetic results. However, saline implants, especially in thin patients with small breasts and minimal fatty tissue on the chest wall, have a much better, softer appearance if the implant is placed below the pectoralis muscle because the implant is covered by a layer of muscle.

Proponents of submuscular placement also believe that the complication of capsular contracture is less likely to occur and that there is less interference with mammogram reading. However, the scientific data on these two points are inconclusive. The current generation of silicone implants that leak less than older models did is expected to greatly reduce the risk of capsular contracture regardless of implant location. Further, the improved ability to more easily read a mammogram is more theoretical than proven.

In patients who have adequate chest-wall soft tissue, submammary placement of the implant may be preferable if the breasts sag. Submammary placement is frequently necessary in extremely muscular patients, such as body builders, because contracture of the pectoralis muscle may severely deform the implant (animation deformity).

The Procedure

Breast augmentation may be done under general anesthesia or with sedation and local anesthesia. It is usually performed in an outpatient setting. The operation takes one to two hours. After making the incision, the surgeon will lift the breast, either below the breast tissue or below the pectoralis major fascia or muscle, as described above, creating the pocket of the desired size and shape. Then the surgeon will position the breast implant (and fill a saline implant) and close the incision with sutures. Steri-Strips, which are small surgical tapes, may be placed over the stitches. The breasts are dressed with a dry dressing and a surgical bra or bandage wrapped around the body. On rare occasions, the surgeon may deem it necessary to place a drainage tube to remove any blood or fluid from the breast-implant pocket.

Recovery

After a recovery time of several hours, patients are typically ready to go home. There may be significant pain and discomfort in the initial hours or days after surgery, requiring prescribed pain medication. Pain usually subsides within forty-eight hours, and after four to five days, most patients are fully active. Muscle relaxants are helpful with submuscular position. Opinions vary on garments to wear after surgery. Some prefer tube tops, sports bras, ACE wraps, or other forms of compression, while others avoid garments that provide external pressure. The breast pain and swelling will rapidly subside within several days and will totally resolve after three to five weeks. Patients should avoid driving and lifting for one week and should gradually increase activities. Strenuous physical exercise should be avoided for at least three weeks.

Sutures are removed after ten to fourteen days. Scars will stay red for at least three months; they then begin to soften and fade. Scars usually will become inconspicuous and cosmetically acceptable. Very rarely, a patient will develop an abnormally thick, ropy scar referred to as a hypertrophic scar or a keloid. If this does occur, these scars will need to be treated with cortisone injections, scar creams, and compression under sheets of silicone. It will take several weeks before a patient is able to see and appreciate the final result of her breast augmentation.

Complications

Although most patients have a successful outcome, there are potential risks and complications. Within the first ten years after surgery, 25% of all augmentation procedures are revised. Possible complications following augmentation are detailed below.

Capsular Contracture

Capsular contracture, the most common complication of breast implants, occurs when scar tissue forms around any foreign body or implant, forming a capsule. Capsular contracture has grades of severity, as shown in the box. If the scar tissue or capsule around a breast implant contracts, it can distort the underlying breast implant and cause a hard, uncomfortable, asymmetric, or rippled breast. Submuscular placement of breast implants reduces the risk of capsular contracture. If significant contracture develops, the capsule may need to be surgically corrected.

Leak or Rupture

Implants are manufactured devices and can experience occasional mechanical failure. The failure rate is around 1% per year, higher in saline

Grade I:	A soft, normal-appearing breast.
Grade II:	The breast is mildly firm to the touch, but no visible abnormality is apparent.
Grade III:	The breast feels hard to the touch, and there is some visual distortion, usually rippling.
Grade IV:	The breast is hard and painful, with marked visual distortion.

and less in silicone. Leaks are evident in different ways. If a saline implant leaks, the leak is usually readily apparent. The salt water leaks and is absorbed by the body, and the implant immediately shrinks. A leak from a silicone gel-filled implant may be subtler. The surrounding capsule of soft tissue that the body creates around an implant will usually contain the leak, although the silicone can leak through breaches in the capsule into the surrounding breast tissue. This can cause the leak to appear some time after it occurs. Free silicone gel may be difficult to completely remove and will calcify because of an immune system response to it. Silicone implants leak more rarely, but when they do, there can be a silent rupture, undetected until the body reacts to the silicone by attempting to encapsulate. A silicone leak may be evident on a mammogram, but taking a mammogram is not advised for younger women. Magnetic resonance imaging (MRI) is the best imaging technique available to detect leakage from an implant. The FDA recommends that patients receiving silicone implants have an MRI at three years after implantation and, thereafter, every two years. However, this is an expensive test, not covered by insurance, and sometimes recast a leak when there is not one. For these reasons, many patients and many plastic surgeons do not follow these recommendations.

Obscuring of Mammograms

A breast implant may compress or overlap surrounding breast tissue, making it more difficult for a physician to read and interpret portions of a mammogram. This is theoretically less problematic with submuscular breast augmentation. Special mammography views and ultrasound may be required to fully evaluate the breast. And while certain parts of the breast are harder to see, other parts are easier to see due to projection away from the chest wall. If mammograms are performed in a radiology center with ample experience with patients who have breast implants, the mammographer can generally interpret the x-ray without much difficulty.

Infection

Infection after breast augmentation is quite rare. If there is an infection localized to the incision, it may be treated with local wound care and antibiotics. If the infection extends into the implant capsule, the implant may need to be removed and replaced later. Although infection may occur months or even years after placement of the implant, infections typically occur within the first five to fourteen days.

Bleeding and Hematoma

If there is bleeding around the implant, it will appear within several hours to days after the operation. The breasts will become swollen and bruised, perhaps requiring reoperation to remove old blood and control any bleeding points. Even moderate amounts of undrained blood can lead to infection and capsular contracture.

Changes in Nipple Sensation or Function

Nipple numbness and extreme sensitivity are both unlikely but potential complications of breast-augmentation surgery. They have been reported in as many as 15% of cases across all incisions and techniques used. Long-term altered sensibility is slightly more common with the periareolar approaches, discussed under "Options for Incisions" above. Normal sensation will usually return to the nipples with time. In rare instances, the abnormal sensation may be permanent.

Changes in Breast Characteristics

Breast augmentation's underlying goal is to change the appearance of the breasts, usually by enlarging or lifting. However, additional breast modifications may occur, whether intentionally or not. These include adjustment of breast position, raising or lowering the inframammary fold, and increasing or decreasing distance between the breasts, which affects cleavage. Some changes may be desired, while others may reduce attractiveness of the breasts by causing asymmetry or malposition. These cases may require another operation soon after the first to correct problems.

Delayed Reoperation

Even with good results, the durability of breast augmentation is about ten to fifteen years. After this time, most patients require reoperation because of leaking, capsular contracture, breast sagging, desired size change or explantation, or implant migration.

BREAST RECONSTRUCTION
AFTER MASTECTOMY

Most women with breast cancer can be treated with removal of the breast lump (lumpectomy) and radiation treatment after surgery. About 30% of women with breast cancer cannot be treated with a lumpectomy and will require removal of the entire breast (mastectomy). Despite the technical advances in breast surgery, a mastectomy results in a significant deformity on the chest wall. The deformity is not just a physical change: a woman has emotional feelings about her loss of one or both breasts. There are important psychological benefits to breast reconstruction for women who desire it.

Clearly, the primary goal in managing breast cancer is cure of the disease. Planning the operation for a cosmetically attractive outcome requires a team of surgeons, so any woman who is about to undergo surgery for breast cancer may consult a plastic surgeon before her surgery if she wishes to have the breast reconstructed. Today, one of every five to six women chooses to undergo breast reconstruction after mastectomy.

Timing and Goals of Reconstruction

Breast reconstruction is done in stages and may begin either at the time of mastectomy surgery or secondarily, meaning, once the incisions have healed and the chest-wall swelling has diminished. Immediate reconstruction is best in most situations; the skin and chest-wall tissues are soft and pliable because there has been no opportunity for scars to develop. But surgeons will usually delay reconstruction under two circumstances: (1) if there is any question about whether the entire tumor has been removed or (2) if they are aware that a patient will need radiation after surgery. Patients should be aware that the surgeon may need to change any earlier decisions during the mastectomy procedure for unexpected findings. Unlike with radiation therapy, immediate breast reconstruction does not interfere with any plans for chemotherapy.

Reconstructive goals are to create a breast mound of size, position, and symmetry that matches the opposite breast. Delayed reconstruction should alleviate any tight scarring on the chest wall, while immediate reconstruction should keep this tension from developing at all. The reconstruction should give the chest a natural female contour so that the patient can enjoy all aspects of life without the worry and inconvenience of wearing an external prosthesis (usually a custom-made bra). The final goal will be to reestablish the nipple and areola.

Options for Reconstruction

There are two general approaches to reconstructing the breasts. The first is to reconstruct the breast with a breast implant. The second is to reconstruct the breast by transferring the patient's own body tissues from another location, that is, by using autologous tissue. To determine how best to reconstruct the chest wall, the surgeon will evaluate the chest skin's quality, the condition of the underlying chest muscles, the amount of subcutaneous fat, the areas of skin laxity, any previous surgical scars on the breast and elsewhere, and—most importantly—the size, shape, and position of the opposite breast.

If the reconstructed breast cannot be made symmetrical with the opposite breast, surgery on the healthy opposite side may be necessary. The options for surgery on the healthy breast include reducing its size (reduction mammoplasty), increasing its size (augmentation mammoplasty), lifting (mastopexy), and removing and reconstructing it (prophylactic mastectomy).

Opposite-breast surgery can sometimes be done when the removed breast is reconstructed, but it is often better to delay the procedure to allow the surgeon to match the final appearance of the reconstructed breast. In 1999, the government legislated that insurance companies who cover breast reconstruction must also cover correction of the opposite breast if such surgery must be done to achieve symmetry.

The decision to operate on the healthy breast must be made very carefully after due consultation with both the plastic surgeon and the oncologist. A woman who has had cancer in one breast has a slightly increased risk of breast cancer on the other side. Therefore, oncologists must feel comfortable about being able to routinely examine the opposite breast in the future, after it has been operated on. Even though examining the healthy breast can be somewhat more difficult after an operation, operating on that breast in no way changes or increases its risk of future cancer. Lately, there has been a strong move toward prophylactic mastectomy and reconstructing both sides the same way.

Reconstruction with an Implant

After a breast is removed, it is difficult to reconstruct a sufficient breast mound simply by placing a breast implant. Fortunately, soft tissues can be encouraged to grow by stretching them, much as some people gradually force larger spaces in earlobes by wearing wider or heavier earrings. Muscles and other soft tissues—even bones—can grow in response to steady pressure from an implant. Any woman who has experienced the stretching skin and muscles of the abdomen during pregnancy knows this remarkable ability of tissue to expand.

At first, a reinforced and externally inflatable implant called a tissue expander is needed. There are several types of tissue expanders, but all have a valve or valves, which can be used later to fill the expander with fluid during an office visit. Some valves are in the wall of the main implant, while others lie under the skin and are attached by tubing to the implant. The valves can be felt through the skin if the remaining soft tissue is thin, but typically, a magnet is used to find the metal back wall of the valve. Occasionally, the expander will be partially filled, or inflated, in the operating room immediately after its placement.

Two-Stage Reconstruction

Placement of the expander is a straightforward operation taking about 1 to 1.5 hours per side. It should not prolong the hospitalization or recuperation significantly after a mastectomy.

Stage 1: Procedure, Options, and Recovery

Reconstruction with an implant must allow time for tissues to stretch, so it is often done in two stages. A tissue expander is placed under the muscles of the chest wall either immediately (at the time of mastectomy) or secondarily (three or more months after the breast has been removed). The muscles and skin are then stitched closed over this relatively empty, silicone-walled balloon. Some surgeons believe that completely covering the implant with both muscle and skin improves results, so they elevate the pectoralis and serratus muscles. Other surgeons leave the serratus muscle undisturbed, as is common with breast augmentation, and cover only a portion of the expander with the pectoralis muscle, largely to hold it in place. Sometimes tissues are added as a support or internal bra or sling to secure the position of the expander and implant. These are typically biologic products made from human or animal tissues.

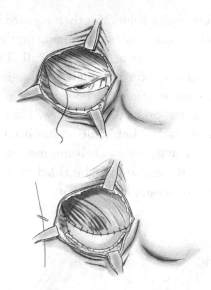

Figure 49: Placement of ADM as internal bra or sling

During mastectomy and placement of a tissue expander, the surgeon will place drainage tubes to drain any blood and fluid that collects under the incision. These drains will be removed between five and ten days after surgery, in most cases, longer with a biologic sling. Stitches are removed between eight and fourteen days. It should take three weeks to resume light activity and six weeks to resume more normal activities.

If the expander is placed as a secondary reconstruction, it is done on an outpatient basis or with an overnight stay in the hospital. It can be done with local anesthesia and heavy sedation, although most surgeons prefer to do the procedure under general anesthesia. Drainage tubes may be placed after the operation, and stitches are removed between eight and fourteen days. Light activity may be resumed within seven to ten days. Normal activities will probably be possible within about three weeks.

Expansion Phase

Patients typically tolerate expansion very well. During each expansion in the clinic office, the skin over the valve will be cleansed with an antiseptic solution. A needle stick will be felt as the needle is passed through the skin to enter the implant's valve. If the patient is sensitive to the needle stick, an anesthetic agent can be applied to the skin forty-five minutes beforehand to minimize discomfort. Saline solution is then injected into the implant. As the solution passes from the valve into the implant, the expander enlarges, stretching the overlying tissues of the chest wall. The expander will be inflated until the overlying skin and muscle feel tight. If it feels too tight or uncomfortable, some solution can be withdrawn. The entire process takes five to ten minutes. Some discomfort will last for one to two days and depends on how much saline solution has been introduced into the expander. Muscle relaxants, such as valium, may ease the expansion. At each subsequent visit, the implant will be filled to larger volumes, further stretching the overlying tissues lying over it.

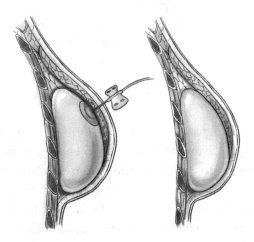

Figure 50: Expansion and then replacement with implant

With both immediate and delayed placement of the expander, expansion typically begins a few weeks after sutures are removed from the incision. It continues every week or two until the chest wall soft tissues have stretched enough to allow a permanent implant to be placed. As a rule of thumb, the expander is inflated 10–25% greater than the desired volume of the final implant. As mentioned above, this process can take several months, depending on the soft-tissue envelope around the expander.

Stage 2: Procedure and Options

In the second operation, the expander is removed, and the permanent breast implant is placed. Modification of the reconstructed breast can also be performed at this procedure. This second operation will usually take 1 to 1.5 hours. In this operation, great care will be taken to match the reconstructed breast with the opposite breast. This is also the appropriate time to undergo any surgery to modify the healthy opposite breast. These operations, unless extensive, can be done as outpatient procedures.

The permanent implants are the same as those discussed in the chapter on breast augmentation. The implants all have walls of silicone and are filled either with silicone gel, cohesive gel, or saline solution. Silicone implants are more predictable than saline-filled implants in providing an aesthetic breast reconstruction. The latter tend to have a tighter, less natural appearance and show ripples.

The implant's silicone wall will be either textured or smooth. Surgeons who favor the textured implants believe that these implants encourage the body to produce less of the tight scar tissue that causes a complication known as capsular contracture. Surgeons who prefer smooth-walled implants believe that these implants give a less rippled appearance to the reconstructed breast and move more naturally. Cohesive silicone implants and anatomically teardrop-shaped implants provide more options for optimizing the appearance and symmetry of a reconstructed breast.

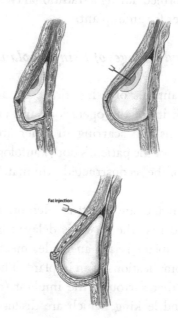

Figure 51: Expansion and then replacement with implant with fat grafting

One-Stage Reconstruction

One-stage implant reconstruction means that the permanent implant is placed at the first stage, which is usually only an option with immediate breast reconstruction while skin laxity is present. An alternate approach uses a combination implant: an inflatable expander that is also a permanent implant. The valve, which is connected by tubing to the implant, is placed near the skin in a location that is both easy to feel and to reach with a needle. Again, the patient will return to the clinic every week or two, and the surgeon will inject saline solution through the valve into the implant. Once the desired volume has been achieved, the valve can be removed in a quick, simple procedure done in the office on an outpatient basis. To remove the valve, the skin lying over it will be sterilized and numbed with a local anesthetic. A small incision is made over the valve, which is pulled free from the implant and discarded. The small incision is closed, with stitches, which will result in a small scar. Although the main idea of using a combination implant is to avoid further surgery, it is important to remember that a second surgery may still be required if it becomes necessary to modify the reconstructed breast position, size, or shape, a step that is commonly performed during a traditional two-stage procedure that exchanges the expander for an implant.

Advantages and Disadvantages of Using Implants

The primary advantages of using tissue expansion and the breast implant are the simplicity of the operations and avoidance of the more complex reconstructions and scarring in other areas that move donor tissues from other parts of the patient's body (autologous tissues). Further, the color and texture of the reconstructed skin matches because expanded skin is chest skin.

The main disadvantages are that this often produces an overly round, less natural breast and that the result is delayed by several months. In addition, the breast implant is a man-made, mechanical device that is subject to any of the complications of an implant. These include tightening of the body's tissues that surround the implant (capsular contracture), rupture, migration, and leaking, which are discussed more fully in the chapter on breast augmentation. Other disadvantages are the needs for multiple office visits during the months of expansion and for two operations unless an expandable or permanent implant is used.

Recalling that cancer treatment is the goal, patients must understand that radiation for control of cancer does change normal chest tissue and that subsequently tissue expansion and implant reconstruction is more complicated in half of all patients who have received or will receive radiation therapy to the chest.

Reconstruction with Autologous (One's Own) Tissues

Reconstruction can be designed to create a breast by moving tissue from another part of the body, where the tissues being moved are commonly referred to as flaps. Choosing reconstruction with a flap may be a matter of preference for the patient or surgeon; flap surgery may be a necessary option when chest-wall skin or musculature is inadequate because of trauma, surgeries, or radiation therapy.

The primary advantages of using flaps are that it provides the most cosmetic and natural breast reconstruction in women with suitable tissue. Because there may not be a permanent implant, some of the potential complications previously discussed for breast implants are avoided. Several surgical methods for flaps are available, but regardless of the method used, tissues transferred onto the chest wall can create a very natural-looking breast with similar skin quality, color, and texture. The size, shape, and appearance of the opposite breast are also more easily matched with a flap. Because a flap allows the surgeon to reconstruct a larger breast with a more natural hang, a patient is more likely to avoid needing surgery on the healthy opposite breast.

The Anatomy of a Flap

The first question of any patient considering this surgery may be the site of the donor tissue. To understand more about the options, some basic information about surgical anatomy is needed. The flap consists of skin, subcutaneous fat, and part of the muscle below them. A muscle is surrounded by a layer of tough tissue called fascia that shapes not only a muscle but also the patient's figure itself. At the mastectomy site, a breast can be sculpted from skin, fat, and any other transferred tissues.

Two types of flaps may be used, and the most important distinction between them is their source of blood supply after surgery. Free flaps are wholly removed from donor sites with their major blood vessels and then placed on the chest with a new blood supply to reconstruct the breast. Other flaps are left attached to blood vessels and other tissues at one edge of the donor site; the attached portion is the pedicle, so these are called pedicled flaps. With any flap, the blood supply must be sufficient to ensure donor tissue's survival as a reconstructed breast.

Each type has advantages and disadvantages in reconstructing the breast. The pedicled flap remains attached to its original blood vessels but less robust blood supply to the flap. Some patients have conditions that prevent use of the pedicled flap; these are discussed under "Complications" below.

Free-flap reconstruction is a complex surgery in which the artery and vein supplying the flap's blood vessels are cut and the flap removed from the body to be taken up to the chest wall. The surgeon then uses a microscope to reconnect the arteries and veins to arteries and veins in the armpit or beneath the ribs with fine sutures. This added complexity adds time and risks but usually involves a two-team surgical approach working on the separate sites in order to limit operative time. After successful surgery, the blood supply is more robust for a free flap than for a pedicled flap, leading to fewer delayed complications. However, failure of the reconnected vessels can lead to complete loss of the flap shortly after surgery. Blood transfusions are not usually required but may occasionally be necessary. Time permitting, a patient can donate her own blood several weeks before surgery so that it can be given during the operation, if necessary.

Surgery with Abdominal Donor Tissue

The TRAM Flaps

The flap most commonly used for breast reconstruction is the pedicled *t*ransverse *r*ectus *a*bdominis *m*yocutaneous (TRAM) flap. The skin and fat of the lower abdominal wall, which are normally discarded in a tummy-tuck operation, are lifted with the abdominal muscles that lie below them. The TRAM's pedicle is the upper portion of the flap, and the flap is rotated through a skin tunnel into the mastectomy site. After considering the size of the breast to be reconstructed and the presence of any scars on the abdomen, the surgeon may transfer tissue from the left, right, or both sides. If the surgeon is concerned about the tissue's chances for survival, an artery called the inferior artery that supplies the TRAM flap can be divided ten to fourteen days before reconstruction with the pedicled TRAM, enough time to allow the superior artery to enlarge; this is referred to as a delay procedure.

The free TRAM flap, which is composed of the skin and fat of the TRAM flap, can be taken with the muscle, depending upon the blood supply in the groin. A very small amount of muscle can be moved with the skin and fat; this is called the muscle-sparing free TRAM flap.

A small percentage of patients may have abdominal-wall weakness or a bulge after a TRAM operation, and some may develop a true abdominal-wall hernia. Fortunately, using synthetic or biological mesh to rebuild the abdominal wall that provided the muscle tissue graft makes this complication far less likely. Mesh is needed to reconstruct the wall because fascia is harvested with the TRAM flap.

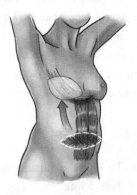

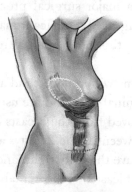

Figure 52: Pedicled TRAM flap

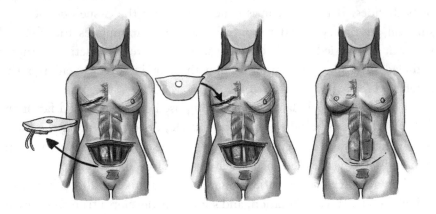

Figure 53: Free TRAM flap

The Free DIEP Flap

Another option is a free perforator flap. All muscle can be spared with the DIEP, deep inferior epigastric perforator flap, or SIEP, superficial inferior epigastric perforator, flap. These are more complicated and longer procedures but may be worth it in certain circumstances. The fascia and muscle are preserved by using a DIEP flap, so using mesh to prevent an abdominal hernia is unnecessary.

The Procedure and Recovery

These flap procedures can be done either immediately (at the time of mastectomy) or secondarily (after some recovery period). The pedicled TRAM operation is a major surgical procedure, and a free TRAM/DIEP operation is a surgery of significant magnitude. A pedicled TRAM procedure can take $2^1/_2$ to 4 hours, and a free TRAM/DIEP procedure can take 4 to 10 hours.

After surgery, drains will remove fluid and blood from the breast, as well as from the abdominal wall, and are usually kept in place for 5 to 10 days. Stitches are removed from the breasts between 10 and 14 days and from the abdomen between 10 and 21 days after surgery. The removal of abdominal skin will leave the belly tight, and the patient will not be able to stand or lie flat for at least a week—remaining bent will minimize pain and avoid tension on the stitches used in the abdominal closure.

This operation requires a prolonged convalescence. Patients usually require a three- to five-day hospital stay. It will take at least three weeks before the patient can resume light activity. It will take about three months for the patient to get back to normal, strenuous levels of activity. A scar will cross the width of the lower abdomen. This scar will be red and noticeable, but redness should begin to settle down by the third month after surgery and will continue to do so for about a year. Scars on the reconstructed chest wall will improve more quickly.

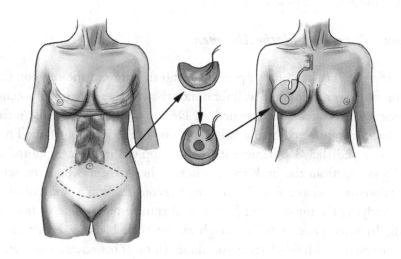

Figure 54: DIEP flap – Muscle left behind

Complications

The major risk of using an abdominal flap, as with any other flap, is that a portion of the flap or the entire flap can die if blood supply is inadequate. This is an unusual complication, occurring in less than 5% of patients. If this necrosis involves skin, it is visible. If fat, a hard area typically develops. The hard area will shrink if it is covered by other tissues, but it may show up as a calcification in mammography exams later.

This complication of tissue loss is more common in patients who smoke cigarettes or who have diabetes, previous abdominal scars, or excessive fat on the abdominal wall. These risk factors may mean any of three decisions: (1) the surgeon must adjust the donor flap site's location on the abdomen, (2) a pedicled TRAM cannot be used because it brings a lower volume of blood to the flap, or (3) either a TRAM with two pedicles or a free flap transfer must be used. Free-flap transfer carries the risk of thrombosis (clotting), where the vessels are stitched together at the site of the reconstructed breast. If clotting occurs, urgent reoperation is needed to prevent complete loss of the flap.

Skin transferred from the abdomen will be numb. It may, over months to years, develop some sensation, but it will be quite different from the normal breast sensation a woman had before mastectomy. As mentioned above, TRAM operations, especially without mesh to replace fascia, can cause abdominal muscle weakness.

Donor Tissues outside the Abdomen

If a patient's anatomy or previous surgeries prevent the surgeon from using the lower abdominal wall for donor tissues, there are other potential donor sites for breast reconstruction. Donor skin, fat, and muscle from the back is transferred on the latissimus dorsi myocutaneous flap. This is usually a pedicled flap because its blood supply is in the armpit and can easily swing from the back to the chest. The latissimus dorsi muscle is occasionally used as a free flap in breast reconstruction as well. Skin and fat overlying the muscle are lifted up and transferred around to the chest wall. In some patients with enough fat on their backs, a breast can be reconstructed with this fatty tissue alone. In most instances, however, the latissimus dorsi myocutaneous flap does require that a patient also have a breast implant to achieve sufficient size and projection. This operation will leave a scar on the back, but the surgeon can often design the operation so that the patient can conceal the scar.

Other areas of the body, commonly the buttock, waist, and outer thigh, can donate free flaps to reconstruct the breast if microscopic blood vessels are found and stitched into their new locations. These depend on the presence of identifiable blood vessels and the amount of fat and excess skin in the donor regions.

Reconstruction of the Nipple and Areola

The nipple and areola are reconstructed only several months after breast reconstruction is complete, allowing the reconstructed breast to settle into its final shape and position. This is a necessary step to take before choosing the location of the new nipple.

There are several ways to reconstruct a nipple. One is to create the nipple with skin flaps from the reconstructed breast. A common procedure of this type is the skate flap, where the skin flaps are shaped like a skate fish, elevated, and rotated to create a nipple papule.

These flaps are designed so that the donor defect (the area where the skin was lifted away) around the nipple is a round, skin-deep incision that is then covered with a skin graft. The skin graft is usually taken from the groin, where the upper inner thigh meets the labia, because this is darker skin that will more naturally mimic the areola. If lighter skin is used, a tattoo can be used to alter the color later. A bolster compressive dressing used to hold the skin graft on the breast will be removed between four and seven days after surgery and must stay clean and dry. The stitches in the inner thigh are removed between ten and fourteen days. Patients usually can get back to light activities within several days, but the incision in the groin may limit activities for several weeks.

A second type of nipple reconstruction is again done with local flaps. In this technique, the nipple is created with a smaller flap from the reconstructed breast, shaped either like a three-pointed star, or a C and two Vs, two ends of an arrow, or one of several other shapes (see figureXXIV-1). The flaps are rotated together to create the nipple papule. The donor sites are stitched together, avoiding the need for a skin graft. Stitches are removed in seven to ten days. Three to six weeks later, the new areola is tattooed with a dye that matches the color of the areola on the other breast. This particular approach is advantageous because the nipple-reconstruction operation can be done with local anesthetic in a short procedure in the clinic. Patients may return to normal activities immediately, although strenuous activities should be avoided for several days. The disadvantage of this approach is that the nipple projection is not as predictable as with the skate flap procedure. Also, the tattooed areola may fade, requiring repeat tattoos after several years.

The third option for nipple reconstruction borrows tissue from the opposite nipple for reconstruction as a graft. If a woman has a long nipple, the tip may be excised and transferred. If a woman has a broad nipple, the lower half can be transferred. This is a composite graft that succeeds only if new blood vessels grow into the graft. Sensation will be absent or very limited.

Other adjunctive procedures may be done during the stages of reconstruction or down the road. This may include modification of the shape, breast fold, size, or skin envelope. One common modification is adding tissue back to the soft-tissue envelope with a local flap or fat grafting (harvested and transferred from the same patient) to add more padding around an implant or into an indention of an autologous flap to improve results.

It is important to know that revisional surgeries are typically every three to five years after breast reconstruction. This is usually based on a patient's choice to modify the shape, size, implant type, or some other feature of the breast for improved cosmesis. However, the complications previously mentioned may lead to a less optional reason for reoperation.

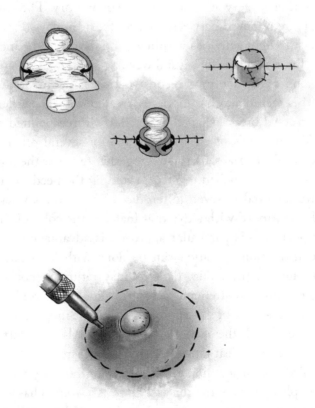

Figure 55: Nipple C-V flap and Areolar Tattooing

RECONSTRUCTIVE SURGERY FOR CONGENITAL BREAST AND CHEST ANOMALIES

Absence of the Breast and Nipple

Congenital absence of the nipple is referred to as athelia. It is very rare to see this deformity on a normally developed breast; it usually is seen when the underlying breast is also absent, a condition called amastia. When a breast gland is absent but a nipple is present, a person has a condition called amazia. These are all rare but troublesome problems. On occasion, absence of the breast can be associated with other chest-wall deformities of the underlying muscles and ribs, as seen in Poland syndrome (discussed below) or other congenital conditions. Amastia can run in families and has also been attributed to some teratogens, which are toxins to which a fetus is exposed before birth. Patients with amastia will usually seek consultation with a plastic surgeon when, or shortly after, the normal breast begins to develop on the other side. It is important to point out that breast development may occur at different rates on each side. Surgery to address the problem should be avoided until it is certain that the missing breast on one side is not simply developmentally delayed. Once an adolescent has enough breast development on the normal side to match, an expandable breast implant can be inserted underneath the skin and/or muscle of the chest wall on the side with amastia. A detailed discussion about these implants and the implantation surgery can be found in the first half of the chapter on breast reconstruction after mastectomy. The patient is seen every few months after surgery for saline to be added into a valve for the implant. This kind of implant can gradually be given enough saline to keep the mound on the amastia side a comparable size to that of the normally developing breast. Once the adolescent has matured, or if the patient is a mature woman when she first consults a plastic surgeon, a permanent breast implant can be placed instead of an expanding one. Tissue donated from elsewhere in the patient's body may also be used, as it is in breast reconstruction after mastectomy. However, the use of donor tissue allows for less adjustment of breast size in the long term, so results may not be ideal.

Breast and Nipple Deformities

Tuberous Breast Deformity

A small percentage of women with underdeveloped (thin and small) breasts may suffer from tuberous breast deformity. The base of the breast is tight and constricted because of a ring of tough tissue called fascia, and the breast seems to bulge out through the constriction. This creates a tubular breast with a large areola around the nipple and an inframammary fold (where the base of the breast meets the lower chest) that is higher than it should be. The problem usually occurs on both sides, but the breasts are not symmetrical.

Correction will usually require several surgeries. The wide areola will need to be reduced, which will result in scars that circle the darker areola where it meets the skin over the rest of the breast. The underlying breast deformity, including surgery to break or disrupt the constricting ring of fascia, can be addressed when the areola is reduced. Unfortunately, the surgeon's ability to see the fascia ring may be limited, and significant dissection of the breast to disrupt the fascia may also disrupt blood vessels that supply the nipple.

To reconstruct the underdeveloped breast, the surgeon may rearrange nearby tissue or use a permanent or expandable breast implant. If a second surgery is necessary, the locations of scars depend on the surgical technique used. Scars from reconstruction with permanent and expandable implants can usually be hidden in the fold beneath the breast. Making an incision here allows the surgeon enough room to modify the breast's shape and move the fold below the breast, which is usually elevated, downward on the chest. Expandable implants are useful in patients who have a breast on the other side that is still developing. Moving donor tissues from other parts of the body creates more scars but can help smooth out the overall breast shape when more severe deformities are present. The surgical details, recovery, risks, and complications are similar to those discussed in "Breast Reconstruction."

Inverted Nipples

Women with otherwise well-formed breasts may have flat or even inverted nipples because the underlying ducts are too short and they "tether" the nipple to deeper breast tissue. Another cause can be having too little tissue bulk under the nipple. In many countries outside the United States, a suction device is available over the counter that provides short-term correction. The apparatus consists of a small cup attached by tubing to a small syringe. When the plunger is pulled outward through the syringe body, suction is created, drawing the nipple outward. The device is left in place for several minutes, three times a day.

There are several operations designed to correct inverted nipples, but these operations will impair and possibly prohibit one's ability to breast-feed a child. The surgery requires making incisions in the skin of the areola and dividing or cutting the tethering ducts. It is helpful to implant something to avoid the nipple from reinverting such as a graft of fat or skin and fat or another type of implant. The scars in the areola are generally acceptable. It is unusual to have any long-term problems with nipple sensation or survival. Inverted-nipple procedures are done with local anesthesia. Sutures are removed in seven to ten days, and recuperation is minimal.

Enlarged Nipples

Enlarged nipples, in the form of long or broad (wide) nipples, may be surgically corrected. It can run in some families, usually becoming more noticeable after pregnancy. Operations to reduce the size of the nipple include removing the tip of a long nipple or removing part of the circumference of broad nipples. Removing the extra width of a broad nipple requires incisions to be closed with sutures. These incisions and their scars can be quite well hidden in the nipple tissue. When removing the tip of a long nipple, the remaining nipple may be closed with sutures or left to heal on its own, which usually allows milk ducts to remain open for possible future breast-feeding. However, any surgery around the nipple can interfere with nursing in women who later bear children.

Congenital Chest Deformities

Poland Syndrome

Patients with Poland syndrome have either absent or underdeveloped muscles of the chest (hypoplasia). This shows especially where one side of the pectoralis major muscle meets the sternum (breastbone) and ribs. One-third of patients have breast abnormalities and defects of the upper ribs, arm, and hand on the same side. The fold in the front of the armpit is usually missing because the pectoralis muscles are not properly developed. The cause of Poland syndrome is unclear, but it occurs during growth and development; it may be caused by an inadequate blood supply. It usually occurs randomly but occasionally runs in families. Patients are usually fully able to move and function normally, but severe forms may impair use of the shoulder, arm, and hand. When to time any necessary operations is controversial. Earlier treatment during adolescence can minimize psychological trauma but add additional insults to physical development. In severe cases, surgical treatments may seek to restore function of the arm by stabilizing the chest wall and restoring muscular function. Cosmetic surgeries recontour soft tissue and reconstruct the breast.

Chest Reconstruction

Implants may be used to fill in the underdeveloped ribs, breastbone, collarbone, and muscle. These may be made of prosthetic mesh, but usually, solid silicone implants are used to provide consistency of muscle tissue, rib, and bone. The breast is usually reconstructed with silicone gel or saline, which may be either a separate implant or a two-chambered, custom implant that also has the solid silicone needed for the chest. Custom implants can be developed from a mold or use radiographic imaging to fit each patient precisely; naturally, custom implants offer significant advantages.

Scars from these surgeries are usually approximately 5 to 8 centimeters (or 2 to 3 inches) in length. An overnight stay in the hospital may be necessary. Drains are occasionally used for 3 to 5 days, and stitches are kept in place for 1 to 2 weeks. Recovery is fairly rapid, but strenuous activity is limited for 3 to 4 weeks (see "Breast Reconstruction After Mastectomy"). Another option is to move or relocate muscles from other parts of the body, a strategy that offers many benefits. Flaps are sections of muscles and nearby soft tissues that also have blood vessels from their donor site; readers are encouraged to review the details of flap surgery under "Breast Reconstruction." The muscle that is used most often is the latissimus dorsi from the back (although it may also be poorly developed or absent in Poland syndrome). The flap can remain attached at one side so that it keeps its blood vessels intact—in this technique, the rest of the flap is rotated from its attachment point, called the pedicle. Rotating this muscle from the back can do all the following: provide soft-tissue bulk, reconstruct the fold in the front of the armpit, cover a permanent or expanding implant, and provide functional, moving muscle. One concern is that the muscle may grow much larger in response to exercise, as would any normal muscle.

If the latissimus dorsi muscle is unavailable, muscle may be moved in something called a free flap from elsewhere, but doing this scars a normal area of the body. It also requires a much more complex surgery that involves recreating attachments to blood vessels and nerves. Also, the ability to function with a free flap is usually not as great as with use of the pedicled (attached) latissimus flap. Donor sites include the latissimus dorsi muscle from the opposite side, the rectus abdominis muscle from the abdomen, and the buttock's gluteal muscles.

Transferring functional muscle is a large surgery that requires a stay of multiple days in the hospital for pain control, recuperation, and observation of the incision. The major risks of the surgery are the flap's failure to survive the transfer, infection, and complications at the incision. Drains are usually used to remove extra fluid for several days to two weeks after surgery. Stitches are left in place for one to two weeks. Physical activity will be limited for four to six weeks, and after this, the patient may need physical and occupational therapy to learn to use the rotated muscle effectively.

Poland Syndrome Breast Reconstruction

The best timing for breast reconstruction for patients with Poland syndrome is late adolescence to early adulthood, which gives the normal opposite breast enough time to fully develop. Breast reconstruction alone may be the only surgery necessary in mild cases of Poland syndrome, but in severe cases, the breast is reconstructed after chest reconstruction is complete. As in reconstruction after breast cancer, either flaps of tissue or implants may be used. When functional muscle must be transposed to correct chest deformities, an expanding or permanent implant will still be necessary to reconstruct the breast; the implant should be placed below the transferred muscle. As mentioned above, these procedures, the choices, recovery, and complications are similar to those discussed in "Breast Reconstruction After Mastectomy."

Pectus Excavatum (Funnel Chest)

Pectus excavatum is a depression of the lower central chest, which occurs in less than 1% of the population. The ribs and muscles are usually not affected, but abnormal cartilage growth and development causes the deformity. Mild cases are difficult to see, but severe cases may push the lungs and other deep structures in the chest out of place. Physiological problems are not common, but severe cases may impair lung and cardiac function, which usually cause the patient to be intolerant of exercise. Besides seeing a doctor for a consultation and a physical exam, patients with significant symptoms may need an x-ray, a CT (computed tomography) scan, an electrocardiogram, an ultrasound of the heart and blood vessels, and lung-function tests.

Minimally Invasive Surgery

Patients with mild or no symptoms usually undergo only cosmetic surgery, which creates minimal risk. They may need only reassurance, and adolescent girls and women may be able to camouflage the abnormality with breast augmentation. These surgeries usually use a custom implant that is manufactured with solid silicone from a template made from the external chest shape or from imaging that uses CT. The CT-directed templates are much more precise than the molded ones, but they are considerably more expensive and require the additional cost of the CT.

These implants are placed through small incisions, under the skin and ideally beneath the edges of the pectoralis muscles. The surgery is done on an outpatient basis or with a stay overnight. Recovery is minimal, and sutures are typically removed in one week. Because of the patient's constant motion in this region of the body, the implants are prone to migration (movement away from original placement), infection, erosion of soft tissue, and fluid collections called seromas and hematomas. Drains are typically used for the first few days to remove excess fluid.

Moderately Invasive Surgery

A fairly new technique developed by Dr. Nuss in 1998 uses camera-assisted scopes through both sides of the chest to expose the internal chest and place a bar below the sternum (breastbone). This bar, when rotated into position, lifts the sternum, correcting the abnormality. The bar is removed two years later.

The procedure's major risks come from making deep incisions into the chest and from elevating the sternum without the surgeon's ability to fully see the lungs, heart, and great blood vessels of the body, which if damaged could cause life-threatening injury. The bar can cause inflammation and even infection of the lining of the lung and heart. This procedure, though less invasive to the chest, has been associated with increased pain, longer hospitalization, and greater risk than the more invasive procedures discussed next.

Highly Invasive Surgery

Procedures to rebuild and reshape the chest are highly invasive. They will impair a patient's future growth, so they should be delayed until late adolescence. One technique is to reshape rib cartilages and correct the sternum by fracturing the bone. The procedure requires large incisions along the sternum (as seen for open-heart surgery) or below the sternum. The bone is stabilized with metal struts, metal plates, reabsorbable plates, metal pins and wires, mesh, or grafts from the ribs.

This major procedure requires multiple hours of surgery, and the patient is usually observed in the intensive care unit (ICU) overnight and in the hospital for one to three days. Drains are placed to remove excess fluid, and the drains and sutures are left in place for one to two weeks. The major risks are damage to lungs, heart, or great vessels, but because the wide exposure of the chest allows the surgeon to see more, these risks are actually lower than with the less invasive, scope-assisted procedure developed by Dr. Nuss. If metal struts were used, they must be removed in approximately six months, but the other materials do not need to be removed.

Pectus Carinatum (Pigeon Chest)

Pectus carinatum is the opposite of pectus excavatum. It is characterized by an abnormal elevation of the sternum (breastbone), is rarer than pectus excavatum, occurs mainly in men and boys, and again has no clear cause. It usually presents in early adolescence as a cosmetic concern with little to no functional impairment. Surgical correction is modified from the invasive procedure just above and has similar treatment planning, recovery, and risks.

Introduction to
Body Recontouring

Many people are not pleased with their current body shape, whether in small or large areas of the body. For concerns about the body's shape, or contour, plastic surgery allows for body recontouring. Some patients consult plastic surgeons about having too much body tissue where they do not want it, while others seek implantation for areas that they feel are lacking.

The complaints that require body-recontouring procedures include generalized fat, localized fatty deposits, excess skin and subcutaneous tissue, or cellulite that causes dimpling and indentations immediately beneath the skin (see figures 56 and 57). Most of the generalized fat on the body is found between the abdomen and the knees, but the arms and back between the shoulder blades are also common areas of concern. Most disproportionately fatty areas involve the abdomen, buttocks, saddlebags, insides of the thighs, and areas above the knees.

In order to correct body-contouring complaints, it is important to define the problem and in simplistic terms: the problem can be excess skin, excess fat, muscle laxity, or loss of volume. By defining the problem, the correct solution can be applied. Excess skin may be tightened either surgically or with skin-tightening technologies. Excess fat can be destroyed, suctioned, or resected. Muscle laxity can be tightened. Volume loss can be replaced with implants or fillers such as fat.

Contour deformities can also result when a person does not have enough soft tissue and fat in localized areas. A small area with a relative lack of projection can be corrected with fat injection. Prefabricated solid silicone implants may be used to augment a part of the body that does not project sufficiently or that has a deficient contour. The most common example is breast augmentation, but the buttocks are also a common area of concern, especially in women. The pectoral region of the chest and the calves are the most common concerns in men.

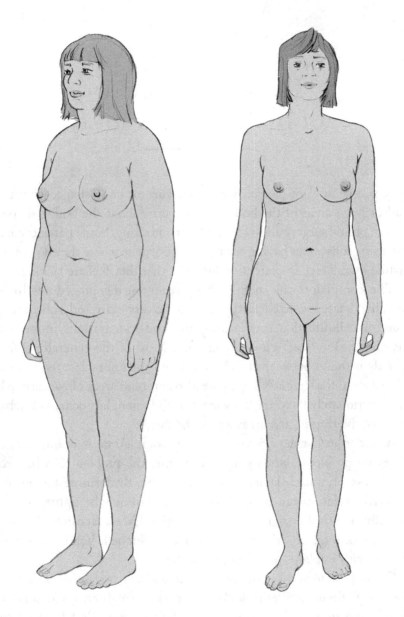

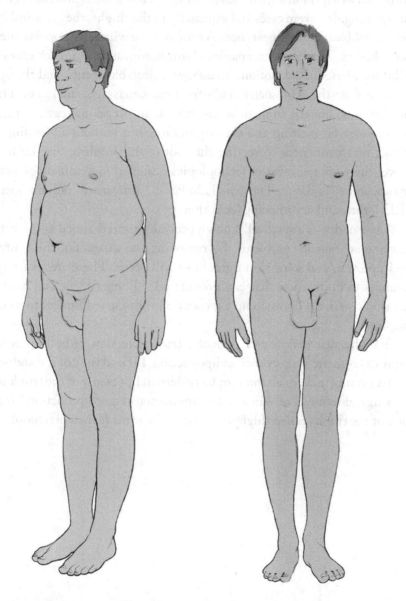

**Figures 56 and 57: Images of general obesity with fat deposits and excess
skin of female and male on left with desired appearance on right.**

Cellulite results in dimpling caused by fat overgrowth between tough bands of tissue (septae) between the skin and the deeper muscles—one may think of it as a quilt in which the stitching is a tissue band and the fat is the soft quilting. In severe cases and especially in the thighs, the areas involved have a cobblestoned appearance. As anyone viewing the popular media today knows, numerous companies claim noninvasive cures for excessive cellulite. These include lotions, massages, injectable agents, and therapies that penetrate the skin, such as radiofrequency, massage, and lasers. There may be some benefit from these treatments in occasional cases typically due to some fat melting and skin tightening, but without addressing the septae, no treatment is correcting the root of the problem. Similar to the above, there are noninvasive technologies designed to eliminate excess fat or subcutaneous tissue. These include lasers, ultrasound, radiofrequency, LED lights, and cryotherapy (cold therapy).

Liposuction is a very well-known procedure and is aimed at correcting excess subcutaneous problems. By removing the excess fat, the contours are improved, and some skin tightening will occur. There are a variety of adjuncts to liposuction that can provide added benefit, such as laser- or ultrasonic-assisted liposuction. Liposuction is discussed further in its own chapter.

For the vast majority of patients, true correction of body problems requires cosmetic surgery such as liposuction, lift and tuck of the abdomen with a tummy tuck, or abdominoplasty dermal lipectomy of the trunk with the surgical removal of skin and fat, augmentation, or liposuction lift and tuck of the thigh (called thighplasty) or of the arms (called brachioplasty).

CELLULITE AND NONSURGICAL LIPOLYSIS

Introduction to Cellulite

Cellulite is a well-known, often discussed, and much hated condition that has always been difficult to treat. Cellulite has three major causes that are necessary for its existence—fibrous septae, fat-cell enlargement, and skin laxity. Fibrous septae, or bands from the skin to the superficial layers of fascia, act as a leash that form the dimples associated with cellulite. These septae typically only exist in female skin leading to the vast prevalence of cellulite in females. As the fat cells in the outer layers of the skin enlarge, they bulge except for where hindered by the septae, increasing the apparent depth of the septae dimples. None of this becomes evident until skin becomes lax enough to allow these contour deformities to show, which is why cellulite shows up later in life.

Treatment is aimed at treating one or more of these three causes—the septae, the excess fat, and skin laxity. Many of the same technologies are adapted in nonsurgical lipolysis as well.

Introduction to Nonsurgical Lipolysis

One of the latest trends in body contouring is the use of nonsurgical device to achieve a reduction in fat and fatty deposits. There are a multitude of technologies aimed at these goals. The key concept is utilizing a technology that leads to controlled injury of the fat cells without causing collateral damage to the skin but preferably with associated skin tightening. The technologies discussed here are external devices. The most common technologies utilized to these ends are radiofrequency, ultrasound, and cryotherapy. Many refer to some of the advanced liposuction techniques such as laser- or ultrasound-assisted liposuction as nonsurgical, but the authors consider these to be surgical and discuss these in the liposuction chapter.

The Technologies

Endermology/Endermologie

Endermology is a technique touted as a nonsurgical procedure to correct superficial bulges cellulite resulting from fatty deposits. The technique has been available for twenty-five years and despite being FDA-approved for this purpose, its efficacy is highly debated. Proponents of the technique believe it works, but most surgeons are unimpressed with the results.

The aim is to provide a firm, toned area with a decrease in superficial fat and the dimpled look that is typical of cellulite. The mechanism uses a handheld device to deliver pulses of electrical heat and massage with rollers applied to areas of cellulite. This combination therapy is suggested to encourage collagen production, fat metabolism, and flow of blood and lymph leading to tightening of the skin and a reduction of the superficial fat. This attempts to address two of the causes of cellulite, but it does not treat the bands. A single treatment lasts between forty-five and ninety minutes, depending on the surface area being treated. The treatment is usually repeated once or twice weekly until the patient is satisfied or until improvement cannot be noted any longer, if it was at all.

This is a nonsurgical procedure without posttreatment discomfort, and regular activities can be resumed immediately. Expense varies, but it is significantly less expensive than the advanced technologies' surgical techniques. Some recommend endermologie as a procedure after liposuction, which is known to benefit from postsurgical massage, regardless of delivery method. The motions and stimulation of endermology are beneficial in this setting.

Radiofrequency

External radiofrequency has more recently been used during attempts to shrink fat deposits, reduce cellulite, and encourage skin contraction. One of the first companies to do so was Thermage, which delivers heat in the form of noninvasive radiofrequency waves to the skin and fat. Other companies have followed suit and all propose to encourage new collagen deposition and dermal skin tightening via the application of unipolar or bipolar radiofrequency. The delivery of radiofrequency energy current is resisted by the tissues, which leads to the buildup of heat, which subsequently leads to some lipolysis (breakdown of fat cells) and collagen remodeling (skin tightening). Results have been inconsistent, and longevity of its effect is unclear, but benefits have been seen. Tolerance is good as the discomfort and downtime are minimal.

External Ultrasound

External ultrasound uses ultrasonic energy applied from outside the body through the skin to cause vibration of targeted molecules, which leads to heat. The heat can lead to collagen damage, which ultimately results in inflammation and the laying down of new collagen, which results in skin tightening. These results are, of course, desirable, but results are inconsistent depending on treatment protocols, depth of skin, skin quality, medications, and health factors. The treatment is mild to moderately painful and duration of effect is limited.

LED light

External LED, or light-emitting diode, uses light energy to change the permeability of the fat cell and allows the contents of the fat cell to drift through the cell membrane, which can then be cleared by the body. The results have been minimal to date, but the technology is being investigated.

External Laser Energy

External laser energy can be used to increase lipase, which can damage the fat cell membrane and lead to its destruction and subsequent clearance by the body. The laser energy has to bypass the skin in order to avoid damaging the skin, which limits the potency of this treatment. The latest technology to the market Sculpsure (registered trademark of cynosure), 1'060 nm diode enery is harnessed with very efficient reduction of subcutaneous fat and some significant skin tightening has been noted. At this time, this seems to be the most effective nonsurgical modality of body contouring.

Cryolipolysis

Cryolipolysis is the application of external cold to the skin to lead to lipolysis, or breakdown of fat cells. Fat is more susceptible to the effects of cold than other tissues, so the ability to destroy fat cells preferentially to other tissues is there, but in order to be safe, the temperatures and time of exposure must be limited, thereby limiting the reduction of fat. Multiple sessions are beneficial, but results can be inconsistent between patients. Pain is minimal.

Mesotherapy

Mesotherapy was originally described in France in 1952 by Dr. Michel Pistor. It involves the injection of a variety of medications to burst and destroy fat cells, whether cellulite or focal fat deposits. The medications are injected with hypodermic needles, and recovery is usually minimal with mild bruising and discomfort. Medications used include vitamins, homeopathic remedies, and pharmaceuticals; there is no regulatory board controlling what products are being injected. There is a risk of allergic reaction to the medication injected, so allergy testing is recommended before treatment. Mesotherapy has not been scientifically proven to be effective, and many complications have been seen.

Although it is minimally invasive, mesotherapy is not without serious risks. Infection can occur. Local structures such as blood vessels, nerves, skin, and tendons can be damaged. Injection into an artery can lead to tissue suffocation and death. Injection into a vein can lead to pulmonary embolism or other lung complications.

The goal of the therapy is the eradication of cellulite or unwanted fat, but when the therapy is excessive, the removal of fat can cause major problems. Cosmetically, the lack of fat under the skin may appear unnatural, uneven, or unhealthy. Functionally, many important structures travel in the fat below the skin. If the fat is removed, this protective and insulating layer is no longer present. For this reason, surgical revision of mesotherapy complications can be extremely difficult and hazardous.

Laser Treatment of Cellulite

The key to any treatment is to address the causes of the disease, and in order to treat cellulite effectively, the physician must treat the septae, the excess fat, and skin laxity. Cynosure developed the first technology that treats all three causes, and it is known as Cellulaze, but other companies are following suit. This device uses laser energy (1,440 nm) subdermally (underneath the skin) in three different directions with an angled laser fiber that is attached to a cannula or fine surgical tube to be manipulated by the surgeon. By lasering down at the skin level, the superficial fat that leads to bulging around the septae is treated and undergoes lipolysis or destruction with melting of the walls of the fat cell. The laser is then used at a cross-cutting angle to divide the septae. Septae have been divided with blades or needles in the past but are prone to heal back together with a sharp incision. The 1,440 nm laser energy melts enough of the bands that they are not in direct contact anymore and, therefore, are less likely to reform. In the third and final stage, the remainder of the laser energy is used aiming at the skin to maximize skin tightening. The treatment is not perfect but attempts to improve all three contributing causes of cellulite.

The procedure may be done awake with local anesthesia or in the operating room sedated, depending on the patient's and surgeon's preference. The swelling and bruising can be significant, but the results have been very promising.

LIPOSUCTION

Liposuction removes fat from undesired areas and other deposits on the body. It was originally practiced in France and has been an accepted procedure in the United States since the early 1980s. The term *liposuction* is used interchangeably for both lipoplasty and suction-assisted lipectomy (SAL). Some recent marketing terms include *liposculpture* and *liposelection*. The body can be sculpted to a more desirable contour by removing undesirable fat, most commonly from the hips, buttocks, knees, abdomen, thighs, back, upper arms, chin, or neck. Some fat may be redistributed, injected, or otherwise modified to augment other areas—lipofilling or fat grafting.

Liposuction was originally developed for individuals with young, tight skin who had disproportionate, localized fat deposits such as in the saddlebag area of the thighs or the love-handle area of the flanks. But with physicians making progressive refinements in the procedure and gaining experience through widespread use over the past twenty years, liposuction is now available to those of all ages and skin types. It can be safe to remove a significant volume of fat from multiple body regions and even to address widespread areas of excess fat. Skin retraction or tightening does occur after fat removal and swelling resolution, but the extent of tightening does vary among individuals, based on genetics, skin quality, age, sun damage, and some unknown factors. Liposuction is not, however, a substitute for weight loss. (See figure 58).

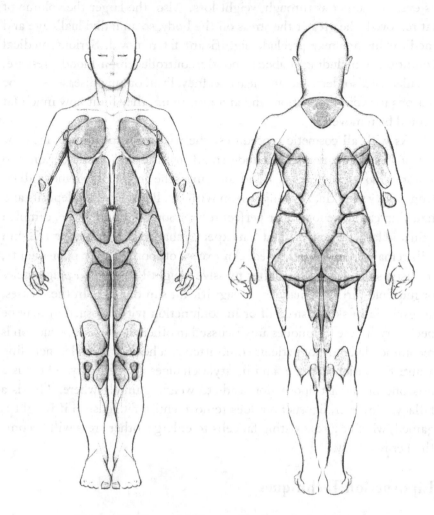

Figure 58. Common Excess Fat deposits locations

The amount of fat that can be safely removed and the ability of the skin to shrink down are limited. With liposuction of a significant volume, the skin is left as an empty bag, not able to contract (tighten) enough as fat is lost. The older the individual, the less elastic the skin, and the less it will recontour after the fat is removed. Also, the overstretching of skin that occurs with massive weight gain and pregnancies reduces the elasticity of skin. Fat lost through dieting and exercise will be lost evenly over the entire surface of the body. Fat removed through liposuction will be more location-specific. Therefore, it is not possible to remove fat through liposuction in as even a manner as through weight loss. Also, the larger the volume of fat removed, the greater the stress on the body, so an individual's age and medical history may preclude significant fat removal. Serious medical conditions—including diabetes, poorly controlled high blood pressure, circulatory disorders, and any heart, kidney, liver, or lung disease—can be reasons to avoid liposuction, and at a minimum, they limit how much fat should be removed.

As with all cosmetic procedures, the patients' expectations must be reasonable, and patients must understand that the goal of liposuction is to restore a more desirable shape and contour to the body, not to remove all fat from below the skin. A young person with small localized fat deposits and taut skin can hope for a near-perfect result. Someone with loose, dimpled skin and larger amounts of fat can expect a change in contour, but the skin will remain loose and dimpled. An excess of loose skin or poor-quality, inelastic skin may be seen after massive weight loss, several pregnancies or multiple-birth pregnancies, or significant sun damage. In these cases, an excision of skin instead of or in conjunction with liposuction may be necessary. These techniques are discussed in other chapters. Liposuction is recommended only for patients committed to a healthy lifestyle, including a nutritious diet, exercise, and lifestyle changes after surgery. There is a misconception that liposuction leads to weight gain elsewhere. This is a fallacy. However, liposuction does remove entire fat cells, so if weight is gained, which causes existing fat cells to enlarge, other areas will become thicker relatively.

Liposuction Techniques

In all liposuction techniques, small incisions are made near the area to be suctioned, preferably hidden in a crease or at least in an area covered by undergarments. A liposuction cannula, one of many metal cylindrical tools of various sizes and shapes, is attached to a suction device and inserted and moved rapidly back and forth to remove fat. Because the cannula tubing is attached to a suctioning apparatus, the desolidified fat is suctioned from the body into a collecting bottle. Each area is usually suctioned from two or more directions in a cross-tunneling technique to obtain a smoother result with less risk of creases and dimples on the skin after healing.

Many techniques are available to suit each patient's needs, and below is a description of each.

- Traditional dry liposuction
- Liposuction with wetting solution
- Power-assisted liposuction
- Ultrasound-assisted liposuction
- Laser-assisted liposuction
- Staged liposuction

Traditional Dry Liposuction

In the dry technique, the liposuction is done on normal tissues without any injections. Both fat and fluids are removed, and approximately one third of the total amount is blood. Blood loss rapidly limits the volume that can be removed, so this traditional technique is practical only for small liposuctions or when harvesting fat for fat injection in another procedure. There is more bruising and risk of irregularities with this technique.

Liposuction with Wetting Solution—Wet, Superwet, and Tumescent

Various wetting solutions can be injected or infiltrated below the skin before liposuction begins. These solutions minimize blood loss, bruising, and pain after surgery, as well as typically containing a crystalloid material, a local anesthetic agent or mixture, and agents that constrict blood vessels. The most common formulation is composed of lactated ringers, lidocaine, and epinephrine, but many surgeons have modified the base formula. The crystalloid material expands fat volume by hydrating the subcutaneous fat layer, making the suctioning easier. The local anesthetic numbs the area during and after surgery. Wetting solutions with local anesthetics allow much higher doses than with direct injection, because the numbing agent is diluted and more slowly absorbed. The agent that constricts the blood vessels, such as epinephrine or phenylephrine, greatly reduces the amount of blood, as well as postoperative ooze and bruising, so that the total amount of blood loss associated with the procedure is minimized and greater volumes of fat can be safely removed.

Greater amounts of wetting improve patients' outcomes. The amount is compared with the amount of fat that the surgeon plans to remove. During wet liposuction, the amount of wetting solution is less than the amount of fat to be removed. In superwet liposuction, the amount of wetting solution is roughly the same amount as the volume of fat to be removed. In tumescent liposuction, a large amount of fluid, typically two to four times as much volume as fat to be removed, is injected into the area. The more wetting solution used, the more space is around the fatty tissue; this allows for more even removal of fat and reduced damage to lymph and blood vessels; using more wetting solution reduces bruising, swelling, and blood loss. Of course, the added step does add time and swelling to the overall surgery, but the larger volumes of local anesthesia used may make general anesthesia or heavy sedation unnecessary. One caution is that, even with slow injection, there is a risk of serious fluid shifts that could cause edema (fluid buildup in areas, including the lungs).

Enhanced Liposuction

Power-Assisted Liposuction

Power-assisted liposuction uses a specialized cannula with movement powered by a mechanical or pneumatic device that assists with breaking up the fat tissue, increasing fat removal with just a standard suction setup. The benefits are that it is less necessary for the surgeon to manually disrupt the fatty tissue and precisely guide the path of the cannula because the motion broadens the effects of each pass. The back-and-forth motions assist in breaking up fibrous fat and larger volumes of fat, and no heat or its negative consequences are generated. It also requires less manual force by the surgeon to perform the procedure.

Ultrasound-Assisted Liposuction

Ultrasonic waves destroy fat cells by causing vibrations that overcome the cell membrane, emulsifying the fat and turning it to liquid. Ultrasound may be applied either internally or externally to assist in liposuction. Internal ultrasound-assisted liposuction (UAL), also referred to as ultrasonic liposuction, transmits ultrasonic vibrations and heat directly to the fat and skin with a specialized cannula used under the skin that is connected to an external ultrasound machine. This makes it easier to remove and allows the body to clear fat cells that are damaged but not removed by surgical tools. In addition, the ultrasonic energy and heat causes beneficial, controlled heat that causes the skin to begin repairing itself by remodeling collagen, which causes contraction (tightening) of the skin.

UAL is particularly beneficial in removing denser, fibrous fat that may be present in a particular patient or in areas that are prone to accumulate dense fat, such as the upper back and the chest wall or breasts in men with gynecomastia. It is also beneficial in liposuctions where scar tissues can make the traditional technique more difficult. Another strong indication for using UAL is in areas of fatty deposits with more significant skin excess. The amount of skin contraction that occurs after UAL cannot be quantified, but experience shows that there is more tightening after its use, and in some cases, it may avoid the need for skin-excision surgery.

UAL is a specialized step that is done after wetting and before suction. Because it is an additional step, the operation will take longer than traditional techniques. The incisions are typically just as well hidden as in the traditional technique, but even with protective efforts, the ultrasonic cannula can cause damage where it enters the skin, leading to delayed healing or a thicker scar.

External ultrasound-assisted liposuction uses ultrasonic energy applied from outside the body, through the skin, making the specialized cannula of the UAL procedure unnecessary. It was developed because surgeons found that in some cases, the direct UAL method increased (1) the risk of skin necrosis (death) when it was used too close to the skin for too much time and (2) the incidence of seromas, which are pockets of fluid under the skin that develop after surgery and cannot be cleared by the body because lymphatic channels were disrupted. External UAL is a possible way to avoid these complications by having the ultrasound applied externally, but it is far less effective. The degree of fat reduction is more dependent on the amount of fat suctioned out with liposuction.

Laser-Assisted Liposuction

Introduced in 2007 by Cynosure as Smartlipo, laser-assisted liposuction (LAL) is another improvement to standard liposuction. As with UAL, it includes an added step between infiltrating the wetting solution and removing the fat by suction. Instead of ultrasonic waves, it uses laser energy to cause lipolysis and skin tightening ("Minimally Invasive Procedures"). The science and options in this arena continue to expand, and many different wavelengths have been used for the procedure. The original lasers utilized 1,064 nm, but it has been found that 520 nm is more effective in coagulating bloods vessels, reducing bleeding, and 1,440 nm is effective at both skin tightening and laser lipolysis. As the power of these machines have increased and the specifics of these procedures have been improved, some dramatic results have been obtained in terms of skin tightening and body contouring. The laser travels through fat below the skin with enough energy to rupture fat cells and cause controlled damage and subsequent contraction of the overlying skin. Laser-energy coagulation also decreases the oozing, bruising, swelling, and recovery versus regular liposuction.

The thinner the tissues and the closer the laser energy can be applied to the skin, the more dramatic the results. Certain areas may only be treated with the laser and no actual liposuction if there is a limited amount of fat present. Common areas for this include the neck and thinner arms. The laser does lyse or rupture the fat cells, and without suctioning, the body is responsible for clearing the damaged cells, which can take several months. Many other companies have entered this arena as competitors with modifications of protocols and laser physics.

Staged Liposuction

Some patients have excessive fatty deposits that cannot be safely removed by excision or liposuction in one session, so subsequent treatments are necessary to achieve the desired result. In an ideal scenario, this situation will be determined before the first procedure so that a patient avoids frustration and disappointment. However, in certain patients, the surgeon may determine during the liposuction procedure that it is no longer safe to remove more fat or that doing so will not achieve the patient's desired appearance. These patients have the option of undergoing another (repeat) liposuction after an appropriate recovery time of several months or undergoing an excisional procedure. This is certainly wiser than putting the patient in harm's way to try to meet expectations. Repeat liposuctions are more difficult to perform because of scar tissue, and due to limits on the ability of the skin to tighten, repeat operations tend to suffer from more intense and prolonged swelling as well skin laxity or dimpling after surgery.

The Procedure

The facility and type of anesthesia used will vary, depending on the surgeon's preference and the amount of fat to be removed. Most liposuction can be safely performed as an outpatient procedure either in the plastic surgeon's office facility or in an outpatient operating room. Small liposuctions can be done using local anesthesia and mild sedation. Medium-volume liposuctions require wetting solutions and sedation. Larger-volume liposuctions require wetting techniques and intravenous sedation, general anesthesia, or regional anesthesia with an epidural or spinal block. When fat is suctioned, the space created temporarily fills with body fluids. These fluid shifts will affect blood pressure, heart rate, and kidney function, so the patient must be monitored carefully during and after the procedure. Volumes of liposuction greater than five liters may require an overnight stay in the hospital or another facility for observation. Some specialized centers perform large-volume liposuction over ten liters, but this adds significant risk and requires meticulous monitoring during and after surgery, fluid replacement through an IV, and possibly blood transfusion.

Liposuction is a technically easy procedure to perform. However, in order to ensure a safe environment and a good result, the procedure should be done in facilities with experience and by physicians who are trained in cosmetic surgery and—even more specifically—in liposuction procedures as it is very easy for irregularities and asymmetries to occur. If heavy sedation, general anesthesia, or epidural/spinal anesthesia is needed, a nurse anesthetist or anesthesiologist is usually present.

Antiseptic skin preparation is more difficult in a treatment that involves multiple areas of the body. It is beneficial to shower the morning of surgery in addition to following the standard recommendations of refraining from eating or drinking for eight hours before surgery. The surgeon will mark the areas and pattern of suction in multiple positions, including with the patient standing up. Preparing the skin with antiseptics may also be done with the patient in a standing position before being placed on the operating-room table. Multiple position changes may also be necessary during surgery.

Most surgeons use either the superwet or tumescent technique, and the use of enhanced treatments with ultrasound or laser is dependent on the patient's preference, the surgeon's preference, finances, availability, and each patient's anatomy. The operation may take anywhere from one hour to multiple hours, depending on the amount of fat to be removed and the number of body sites and positions undergoing treatment. Replacing the lost body fluid with intravenous solution is important in preventing trouble caused by low blood pressure and fluid shifts.

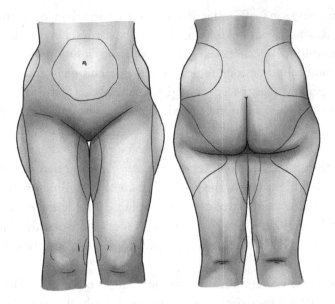

Figure 59. Common areas of disproportionate lipodystrophy

Recovery

After liposuction is completed, the incision may be closed with stitches or tape and then a snug-fitting garment is placed to limit swelling and fluid collection. As the local anesthetic wears off in the hours after surgery, symptoms may include moderate discomfort, stiffness, burning sensations, areas of decreased sensation, or even severe pain that requires prescribed medication. The pain will dissipate after several days and usually resolves within two weeks.

There will be some bloody drainage from the incisions. Significant bleeding is rare, but often the remaining wetting solution continues to drain, and even a slight amount of blood can make the drainage appear bright red. Sutures (stitches) may be removed in a week. Bruising is significant but resolves over one to three weeks. The amount of time needed before returning to work and limited activities depends on individual circumstances but typically ranges between three to ten days. Neither heavy exercise nor strenuous activities should be resumed for four to six weeks.

Depending on skin tone and the volume of fat removed, a compression garment is typically needed for four to six weeks to help the skin recontour and to prevent irregularities such as dimples and creases. Some surgeons prefer continuous use of the garment, whereas others allow removal for showering or allow wearing the garment for only part of the day. Regardless of the precautions taken, significant swelling occurs after surgery and prevents the patients from seeing the results for several weeks before it starts to resolve and some of the benefits can be appreciated. It may take three months for most of the swelling to resolve and six months to disappear completely. A therapeutic massage program, begun after the patient stops using the compression garment, can reduce swelling, help soften scar tissue, and aid in achieving a smoother result. Ideally, this will be done once or twice daily with either direct hand massage or an electronic massager and continued for another four to six weeks.

Complications

Many of the life-threatening complications discussed in the media have occurred in the hands of poorly trained or poorly equipped doctors. These include bowel and blood vessel perforations, nerve injuries, complications related to improper fluid and blood replacement, hypothermia, and infection. These complications can be minimized by a careful choice of a properly trained and certified plastic surgeon and surgical facility.

However, there are potential complications in even the best of hands. These are statistically very unlikely and are treatable if they should occur. They include dehydration, excessive pain, infection, bleeding, poor results, fat embolism, and blood clots that can cause deep vein thrombosis or pulmonary emboli. True dehydration requires oral and, frequently, intravenous fluid replacement. Excessive pain and discomfort may be more severe or prolonged, lasting beyond the initial several days. There are too many variables to determine anticipated pain before surgery. If severe pain is present, it may be caused by low pain tolerance, reduced response to pain medication, infection, hematoma, or damage to nearby structures such as nerves or muscle. When severe pain occurs, a thorough physical exam should determine whether there is a surgically correctable problem. If not, temporary modification of activities or medication may be necessary.

Any surgical incision can develop an infection, and a serious infection characterized by redness, pain, or drainage of pus may require intravenous antibiotics or drainage. Postoperative bleeding is very rare, but stopping it may require operative intervention. As mentioned, liposuction access sites tend to drain bloody fluid for several days, but evaluation by the surgeon is necessary if bleeding is excessive, does not stop with pressure and ice, or is causing a hematoma, pooling collection of blood.

The most serious risks of liposuction that do not depend on the surgeon's technique include fat emboli and thrombosis (clots in the deep veins of the legs or that travel to the lung). Fat embolization may occur at low levels in most liposuction cases. This occurs when fat is delivered to a blood vessel and is transported to an end vessel, where it prevents blood from flowing. Although rare, if this occurs in a large vessel, the patient may develop trouble breathing, a rash of thrombosed or ruptured blood vessels, or a stroke. If deep vein thrombosis occurs, patients may develop asymmetric swelling, shortness of breath, rapid breathing, and decreased oxygenation if a clot travels as an embolus to the lungs. In rare cases where there is a congenital opening between the left and right sides of the heart, it may present as a stroke. Any of these symptoms require urgent evaluation. Embolism is a serious medical condition and requires immediate care, typically with steroids. Thrombosis of the deep veins can occur with any surgery, even with low risk factors and when appropriate preventive measures were taken. Treatment requires anticoagulation, or blood thinning.

Examples of poor cosmetic results include depressions, dimples or creases, irregularities, burns of the skin from laser or ultrasound assistance, residual fat deposits, asymmetry, skin laxity, or recurrence of fat deposits. If too much fat is removed from an area, there can be a local depression, which may be improved by touch-up liposuction around the depression and/or reinjection of fat into the depression. Dimples and creases can be minimized when the surgeon uses cross-tunneling and careful liposuction technique and when the patient uses the compression garment properly and keeps up the proper massage regime. Some dimpling may be unavoidable in individuals with preexisting cellulite, dimpling, or skin laxity. If an area of residual fat deposit is missed or undersuctioned, it is correctable with a repeat, touch-up liposuction. Once fat cells are removed, they cannot be replaced, but the cells left behind retain the ability to store fat. If the patient practices a lifestyle of poor diet and exercise after liposuction is completed, fatty deposits can recur and occur to a greater extent in untreated areas. If it does occur, touch-up liposuction and modification of lifestyle can correct the problem.

Combination of Liposuction with Excisional Procedures

Liposuction is often combined with excisional procedures either at the same time or as a preliminary stage, either planned or unplanned. Most body contouring discussed in the following chapters are improved by adding liposuction to the procedures. There is a limit on how much and where liposuction can occur with these procedures in order to minimize the risk of complications. If the tissues are very thick with fatty tissue, it can be wise to perform liposuction aggressively. This will leave skin laxity that can then be removed in a subsequent procedure with far decreased risk of skin death (necrosis) or problems healing. The skin may be quite lax and appear worse in the interim between the two surgeries, but in the end, more fat is able to be suctioned, and more skin is able to be removed than if the two procedures were done during the same operation. In certain cases, it may be determined after liposuction that excess skin laxity may require an excisional procedure such as a lift or tuck.

ABDOMEN

The abdominal wall consists of skin, the fatty subcutaneous layer beneath the skin, and the muscle layer below. All layers are affected by changes occurring with age, pregnancy, and weight gain or loss. Individuals with reasonably good skin and muscle tone may have excess fat alone, so they may be candidates for corrective liposuction. If correcting the protrusion of the abdomen requires removal and tightening of skin or repair of the weakened abdominal muscles, then a surgical procedure known as an abdominoplasty, or tummy tuck, is required. There are many variants of an abdominoplasty, but the most common ones are a full or standard abdominoplasty, a mini abdominoplasty, a limited abdominoplasty, a lipoabdominoplasty, a reverse abdominoplasty, and a fleur-de-lis abdominoplasty.

Liposuction

If there is excess fat with an appropriate amount of skin with remaining elasticity, liposuction of the abdomen can be performed through very small incisions inside the navel (umbilicus), in a crease in the skin on the lower part of the abdomen, or in the pubic hair area to suction between the ribs and pubic area. The flanks and love handle areas can also be reached from these incisions, but if necessary, an incision is made in a crease in the flank. Liposuction of the abdomen may be done in the abdomen at the same time as in the buttocks, hips, or thighs or with a more invasive surgical procedure. The fat is suctioned by the techniques discussed in its chapter.

Abdominoplasty (Tummy Tuck)

Standard Abdominoplasty

Individuals in reasonably good health with an abdomen that protrudes because of excess fatty tissue, loose skin, and weakened abdominal muscles are ideal candidates for a standard abdominoplasty. These features may occur in patients of many ages, either as a congenital predisposition or because of advancing age or previous pregnancy or surgery. Most women who have had previous pregnancies are candidates for an abdominoplasty for two reasons. The stretched skin of multiple pregnancies often loses elasticity and may not return to its preconception state, resulting in an excess of abdominal wall skin. And as the abdominal wall stretches during pregnancy, the rectus muscles (six-pack abdominal muscles) are splayed apart. If the two vertically oriented rectus muscles remain separated rather than touching in the midline, a diastasis rectus is present. This widens the girth of the abdomen and may allow the contents inside the abdomen to protrude, but it is usually not a true hernia. Cesarean section and other abdominal operations can make a diastasis rectus worse.

An abdominoplasty is a cosmetic operation that is not covered by insurance, but occasionally, abdominal weakness may be associated with an abdominal-wall hernia that needs repair. In these cases, an abdominoplasty may be done at the same time, and part of the procedure may be covered by insurance.

The Procedure

Abdominoplasty with muscle repair will usually require general anesthesia, deep sedation, or an epidural block. If the correction is directed at skin and fat only, intravenous sedation and local anesthesia delivered in a wetting solution like the one used in liposuction may suffice. The operation can be safely performed in an outpatient or office-based operating-room facility. A standard or full abdominoplasty procedure takes approximately two to three hours. Going directly home the day of surgery after recovery from anesthesia is possible, but many surgeons recommend at least overnight observation in the hospital or recovery facility.

Preoperative markings are designed and drawn on the skin when the patient is both standing and in a flat position. An underwear or bathing suit design can be accommodated to hide the scars if the preferred garment is brought to the facility. To remove the excess tissue and tighten the abdominal skin, the incision is large, extending across the abdomen from hipbone to hipbone at about the level of the inguinal crease and pubic hairline. However, it can be hidden under clothes and usually fades nicely. A second incision is needed around the navel, but the navel is preserved.

The abdominal-wall skin and fat are lifted off the muscle below to the level of the ribs. This allows the surgeon to tighten the muscles of the abdominal wall and all the abdominal skin. Ideally, all the excess skin and fat between the navel and the pubic incision is then removed. The separation between the rectus muscles is repaired with stitches that pull the muscles tightly together in the midline from the xiphoid (lower central ribs) to the pubic bone. Second and third rows of stitches may be placed in the muscle layers on each side to recreate a tighter waist. The raised abdominal skin is then pulled down and redraped snugly to the lower incision with tacking sutures. A hole is cut in the abdominal skin where it meets the natural navel, and then the navel is pulled through and sutured into position. Liposuction of the flanks is typically necessary. Drainage tubes are usually placed to remove any fluid and blood that collect beneath the incisions.

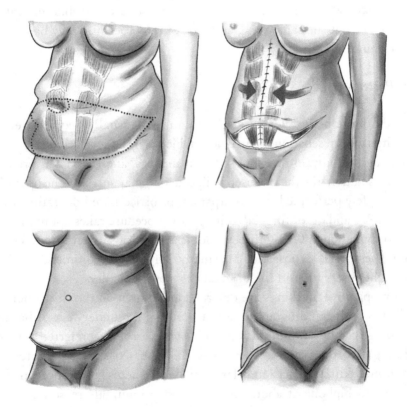

**Figure 60. Basic Steps of Abdominoplasty. 1. Skin removal.
2. Muscle Plication 3. Closure and Liposuction 4. Drain Placement**

In order to maximize the amount of skin removal and cosmetic result, the patient is positioned in a flexed, or bent, position with the legs and back up in a "beach chair position." This takes tension off the stitches, but as the skin stretches over the first week, the patient will be able to stand and lie straight. Finally, all incisions are completely closed with sutures and a dry gauze bandage is applied, typically with a compression garment.

Recovery

An abdominoplasty is a major surgical procedure, and there can be considerable discomfort and pain after surgery, especially in the initial twenty-four to forty-eight hours. Some patients will require intravenous, narcotic pain medication in the initial hours, but oral prescription pain medicine will suffice for most patients after the procedure. Pain subsides slowly over several days, although discomfort, mainly from plicating the rectus abdominis muscles, can last for several weeks. Drains are removed when drainage is minimal, typically by five to ten days after surgery. Stitches are removed between one to two weeks after surgery if nonabsorbable suture is used.

Patients are in a bent position initially, and slowly straighten up within seven to ten days. A compression binder around the body in the initial weeks can limit swelling, but swelling in the lower abdomen will fluctuate with the patient's level of activity for two to three months. Patients usually need at least two weeks before returning to work. Many individuals require three to four weeks to return to normal daily activity, even with restrictions. Strenuous activity, sexual activity, or lifting over twenty pounds should be avoided for six weeks, and heavy exercise should progress slowly between six weeks and three months.

An abdominoplasty is an excellent operation for abdominal-wall recontouring and strengthening of the abdominal wall. Most patients have a drastic overall improvement and sense of well-being with less low-back discomfort and improved strength as a result of the muscle repair. The trade-off is a lower abdominal scar. Initially, the scar will be red, but at three to four months, the scar should start to soften and fade, a process typically completed by twelve to eighteen months after surgery. The scar may widen some due to the tension place at surgery, but staying hunched over to minimize tension is helpful.

Complications

Being a major procedure, standard risks of all operations apply. These include serious risks such as deep vein thrombosis, pulmonary embolism, bleeding, and infection. However, these are extremely rare if the surgeon takes appropriate precautions and chooses patients carefully. Some patients with significant medical problems may be told that they are not a candidate for this elective, cosmetic operation. The most likely, though thankfully still unusual, complications are hematoma, seroma, infection, skin loss (necrosis), scars, and "dog ears." After surgery, if blood collects as a hematoma beneath the abdominal skin, surgery to remove the blood and replace the suction drains for several days is needed. Other fluids that do not contain blood may collect under the skin after the drains are removed (as a seroma). If enough fluid accumulates, it may need to be removed with a needle and syringe; occasionally, drains will need to be replaced for several days.

Infection is rare after an abdominoplasty, but if one should occur, a serious infection could require intravenous antibiotics and surgical drainage of the infection.

Because this surgery elevates the abdominal-wall tissues, a decreased blood supply reaches the abdominal skin. On rare occasions, this can lead to an area of skin or fat necrosis, but this is seen more commonly in patients with other medical problems such as marked obesity, diabetes, or history of cigarette smoking. The skin necrosis may cause the incision to separate or a patch of dead skin and fat in the lower part of the abdomen to form just above the scar. In most cases, the area is small and can be treated with dressing changes. In rare instances, a large area may require surgery revision.

Most scars resolve satisfactorily, but any thickening or elevation of the scar can be treated with cortisone injections and/or pressure dressings made of silicone. "Dog ears" refer to extra skin and fatty tissue at the edges of the scar. This is caused by the ending of the surgical excision adjacent to the area beyond the excision. The surgeon will inevitably leave some "dog ears" to reduce the length of the scar, but most "dog ears" will settle down over several months. If they do not, they can be revised with a second small excisional surgery or liposuction.

Mini Abdominoplasty (Mini Tummy Tuck)

A mini abdominoplasty may be appropriate if the skin excess is mild to moderate and is limited to below the belly button, the fatty deposits are primarily below the navel, and the muscle weakness is either not a problem or is limited to the abdominal wall below the navel. This is a less invasive operation that can be done with sedation and local anesthesia as an outpatient procedure without observation in the hospital after surgery.

The Procedure

A smaller incision is made just above the pubic hairline. The incision length depends upon the amount of excess skin and varies from three to eight inches. The skin and fat are lifted off the abdominal-wall muscles between the low incision and the navel. Vertical muscle weakness in this area can be repaired with stitches. Excess skin and fat is removed from just above the incision, and then the skin is resutured into position above the pubic bone. Suction drains may or may not be needed. A mini abdominoplasty may be performed in conjunction with a liposuction of the abdomen, hips, back, flanks, or any other area. If the upper rectus muscle (above the navel) also has a diastasis (is separated), endoscopic tools can be used to stitch together the muscles above the umbilicus.

Recovery

Recovery is faster for this procedure than for abdominoplasty patients but will still require seven to fourteen days before returning to work. Moderate activities are limited for about three weeks and strenuous activity and exercise for about six weeks. Stitches are removed in one to two weeks. Complications are even less likely than after abdominoplasty, but the same basic problems may occur. The major advantage of the mini abdominoplasty is a significantly shorter scar. As with abdominoplasty, the scar will be red initially but will fade in time.

Limited Abdominoplasty

A limited abdominoplasty lacks a specific definition but is any variant between a mini abdominoplasty and a full abdominoplasty. This may include significant abdominal liposuction with a shorter scar abdominoplasty. If there is some mild to moderate skin laxity above the umbilicus, an abdominoplasty with the release and floating of the umbilicus down a few centimeters with a reattachment may be able to achieve full abdominal improvement without the full length and periumbilical scar of a full abdominoplasty. The final position of the umbilicus must be anticipated for a good result. Another variant would be a full abdominoplasty without muscle repair, which would decrease the recovery.

Reverse Abdominoplasty

In certain patients, excess abdominal tissue needs to be taken from the upper abdomen rather than from the lower abdomen. Reasons for this will be a preexisting scar in the upper abdomen that will limit blood supply to the skin that will be lifted in the standard abdominoplasty or upper abdominal excess that will not respond to standard abdominoplasty. It can also be appropriate when done in combination with a breast procedure, whether by augmenting the breast using the elevated abdominal skin or during a reduction procedure in order to minimize incisions. The incision is placed in the fold below the breasts, but it still tends to be visible, especially in the midline, and distortion of the important inframammary fold is common. For these reasons, this technique is used only selectively. Recovery, complications, and outcome are otherwise similar to those in the other abdominoplasty procedures.

Lipoabdominoplasty

While any type and many abdominoplasties include some liposuction, a lipoabdominoplasty may be recommended when the abdominal tissues are very thick. Aggressive liposuction associated with the lifting and pulling of a standard abdominoplasty can lead to blood-flow problems with subsequent skin or fat necrosis, although tumescent anesthesia makes this far safer in combination. If a patient is in need of extensive liposuction to obtain an acceptable contour, the options are staging two surgeries with a preliminary liposuction followed by an aggressive abdominoplasty two-three months later or to do aggressive liposuction but minimal undermining and less skin removal from the abdomen in order to preserve more blood vessels to the abdominal apron. This modification allows for a large abdomen to be better addressed in one stage but will, of course, be less tight than a standard abdominoplasty. Recovery is typically characterized by a longer period of drain requirement and prolonged swelling.

Fleur-de-Lis Abdominoplasty

The above abdominoplasties focus on vertical skin excess of the abdomen, best represented by folds and pooches on the abdomen above or below the umbilicus. Appropriate selection of an abdominoplasty can correct this, but if there is a significant circumferential laxity represented by vertical ridges or large flank rolls, these can be aggressively addressed with a fleur-de-lis abdominoplasty. This can also be improved with a circumferential body lift or belt lipectomy, which will be addressed in the next chapter. A circumferential body lift can help a person who has lost massive amounts of weight by combining an abdominoplasty, outer-thigh lift, lower-back skin removal, and buttock lift. A fleur-de-lis abdominoplasty includes removal of the lower abdomen as in an abdominoplasty but also removing a semiellipse from the central abdomen vertically, allowing multiple vectors of tightening. The name is derived from the fleur-de-lis shape of the preoperative drawings.

This operation can lead to a dramatic improvement in the body contours. The downsides are the vertical scar that will not be hidden in a two-piece bathing suit, frequently some increased scarring and distortion of the new umbilicus, and an increased risk of wound healing troubles at the upside down T position in the lower abdomen. Due to the incision in the middle, the tips of the flaps have less blood supply than a standard abdominoplasty, and this may lead to some healing troubles. The recovery is a bit more significant than a standard abdominoplasty as more protection (beach chair and hunched over) is necessary to protect the incisions, and swelling is more prolonged due to more incisions. Muscle repair can still be completed as with a standard abdominoplasty.

Conclusions

There are a variety of abdominoplasty procedures that can be tailored to an individual to achieve a dramatic improvement in abdominal contours. Many women are hesitant to proceed with this surgery, but most patients who have completed the surgery and appreciated the changes recommend without reservation and would definitely do it again.

BODY CONTOURING OF THE TORSO/GENITALIA

Torso Procedures for Obesity

Individuals with abdominal laxity because of massive obesity may have a large bulge or a hanging, overlapping apron (pannus) of skin and fat. This overhang can cause significant musculoskeletal stress as well as hygiene issues. Overhanging folds can suffer from persistent moisture with associated wounds and infections, typically yeast. If severe enough, removal may even be covered by insurance as being medically necessary with appropriate documentation of failure of conservative therapy documented by medical doctors—weight loss, anti-inflammatories, and personal hygiene. If it is deemed to be in need of removal by patient and plastic surgeon, the patients and the pannus may be too large or may have too much scarring on the abdominal wall from prior surgeries to undergo an abdominoplasty safely. The lifting and thinning of these large tissues could have significant risk of necrosis, and cosmesis may be severely impaired even with surgery. Such patients may be candidates for abdominal dermal lipectomy, which is also known as a panniculectomy. This functional procedure is excision of the overhanging abdominal pannus without additional tucking or thinning in order to alleviate hygiene and musculoskeletal issues. This can occasionally be complemented with cosmetic adjuncts such as liposuction or abdominoplasty.

Abdominal Dermal Lipectomy, or Panniculectomy

The Procedure

In a panniculectomy, the excess fat and skin is removed from the abdominal wall without raising the rest of the abdominal wall off the muscular layer. The incision is closed, leaving a horizontal scar along the width of the lower abdomen. If the tissues are very loose both across and down the abdomen, the skin and fatty layer may be removed across the lower abdomen and down the midline by a procedure known as a fleur-de-lis panniculectomy. In heavy patients, this is a significant surgical procedure that needs to be performed under general or epidural anesthesia. An overnight stay will be required, and patients often stay in the hospital for two to three days. Suction drains will be placed at the time of surgery; these drains will be removed once the drainage has slowed, sometimes up to two to three weeks after surgery. As with an abdominoplasty, it will usually take three weeks to get back to work and moderate activity and six weeks to get back to more strenuous activity.

Complications

Complications are significantly higher in this group because of the medical problems and hygiene issues that made an abdominoplasty unsafe. To make this surgery safer and less likely to cause life-threatening blood clots in the legs (deep vein thrombosis), patients must improve eating habits before surgery, be motivated to move and exercise more, and control other medical conditions before and after surgery. Delayed healing and incision infection are common surgical complications in obese patients, especially those with chronic panniculitis, infections in the moist folds. This frequently leads to postoperative infection or partial or complete incision separation (dehiscence), which requires prolonged incision care or a secondary procedure to control incision infection or delayed healing. Other potential complications are similar to those described for abdominoplasty, but all are with increased frequency.

The Back

The back is less often in need of recontouring, especially the full surface, but small areas frequently need treatment. In certain patients, an undesired area may need liposuction of fat or skin and fat removal (by dermal lipectomy). These areas of excess on the back are classically located in two locations: the side of the midback below the shoulder blade often an extension from the breast, and the flank area, which may extend above the buttock. These areas tend to be proportional to the remainder of the trunk but often remain and may even be more noticeable after abdominal liposuction or abdominoplasty (or tummy tuck).

Liposuction

Liposuction of the back is appropriate for excess bulk caused by fat under mildly excessive skin with adequate tone. It is important to note that the fat of the back tends to be more dense and firm; furthermore, it tends to be attached to other structures and partitioned or divided by other tissues. Therefore, only extreme effort will ensure even removal of fat from the back. The procedure benefits from assistance with laser, ultrasound, or power-assisted liposuction more so than other areas due to the dense adherence in the area. Local or tumescent (infiltrated fluid) anesthesia is used, and sedation is usually necessary.

Dermal Lipectomy

If there is markedly excess fat or a significant amount of loose, hanging skin that will not be able to contract sufficiently, liposuction will lead to a poor result. Especially beneath the shoulder blades, the removal of large amounts of fat under lax skin will lead to hanging sheets of skin, which can be less desirable than bulky deposits. In these cases, direct removal of skin and fat is helpful, but its benefits must be weighed against the resultant scar that can be difficult to hide.

Dermal lipectomies can be done with sedation and local anesthesia, but some patients require deep sedation or general anesthesia. Designing markings before surgery is vital. The one- to two-hour outpatient operation involves minimal lifting of skin because this is more of a tissue removal than a lift. The incision is sutured in multiple layers from deeper to superficial over a drain to remove excess fluids.

Drains are usually kept for five to seven days and sutures for one to two weeks. Mild to moderate bruising, tenderness, pain, and swelling are expected, and it may take one to two weeks for the majority of these to resolve. Return to work and activity may be delayed between one and six weeks, depending on required activities. Unexpected complications include bleeding, infection, delayed healing, tissue necrosis, seroma (fluid buildup), and disappointing results, as discussed under other book sections on lipectomy.

Circumferential Body Lift (Belt Lipectomy)

A circumferential body lift can help a person with a great excess of skin and fat on the abdomen, back, thighs, and buttocks. The belt lipectomy has become increasingly common because of the large number of patients undergoing gastric bypass surgery. These patients, as well as patients who naturally lose massive weight, have extra skin that droops in an inverted cone shape from the torso with massive excess in the lower trunk that overhangs their genitalia. They have a poorly defined waist and transition from the back to the buttock, making clothing oneself difficult and cosmesis poor. This procedure can result in dramatic reduction in waistline girth, but it typically creates a relatively straight profile. It cannot recreate an hourglass-shaped torso because the skin is hung (suspended) from above. The goals for the surgery are individualized but generally involve eliminating folds and tightening the abdomen while suspending the skin of the buttock, thighs, and pubic area. This major surgery requires the patient to be turned during the operation to provide access to the entire circumference of the torso. It combines an abdominoplasty, outer thigh lift, buttock lift, and lower-back tuck.

As expected, the belt lipectomy carries the risks of each of these combined procedures, and more, because it is harder to be protective of all areas at the same time. Therefore, patients with significant medical problems should not undergo this operation. Drawing good markings and making good plans before surgery are essential, as is having a well-coordinated patient-care team that includes the surgeon, nurses, surgical assistants, and anesthesia providers.

The Procedure

Markings are drawn on the skin to maximize tissue removal on the front and sides rather than on the back. An incision is made around the body, and in the front, the tuck is down with a conservative abdominoplasty, and the lateral thigh is lifted, and on the back, the upper buttock is lifted to the lower back. The separation between the abdominal muscles (rectus diastasus) can be plicated as in an abdominoplasty.

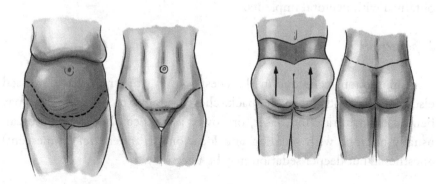

Figure 61. Basic Components of Circumferential Body Lift.
1. Abdominoplasty. 2. Buttock Lift

Recovery and Complications

Recovery can be prolonged, given the significance and frequency of incision-healing issues in this procedure. Using several suction drains is essential. Minor complications are extremely common and include seromas, small infections, and partial wound separations. Major complications such as hematomas, major wounds, and blood clots are possible but unusual.

Patients rest with the hips mildly flexed for one week before slowly straightening. Normal walking and activities of daily living are essential but can be difficult for the first one to two weeks. Exercise and more significant activities should be avoided for four to six weeks. Patients are usually quite pleased with the operation, but it is important to realize that this operation is as functional—to aid daily life—as it is cosmetic. The cosmesis of the tucking and scars will not be as good as if these procedures were done in stages.

The Chest

The chest may also have excess skin or fat, prompting individual patients to consult a plastic surgeon. Liposuction is the most common method used to treat the chest because of the high visibility of scars that would be caused by skin removals and the ability to fade liposuction into untreated areas. In women, this procedure may be combined with cosmetic breast surgery. In men, it may include recontouring of the breasts at the same time, even in men who do not have gynecomastia. Other men may choose the appearance of larger pectoralis major muscles (pecs) that are obtained with pectoral implants.

Liposuction

Liposuction technique in the chest wall is similar to that discussed elsewhere. As with fat in the back, chest fat tends to be dense and may benefit from ultrasound, laser, or power assistance. The procedure can usually be done with sedation and local or infiltrated wet (tumescent) anesthesia, but deeper sedation may be necessary.

Chest Dermal Lipectomy

Unless combined with breast procedures or after weight loss, removing chest tissue by dermal lipectomy is rarely necessary. When combined with breast procedures, the incision can be extended to include chest areas, especially the axillary rolls on the sides near the armpits (see figure XXX-3). It can usually be placed in an existing fold, but because the goal of the surgery is to reduce or eliminate these folds, the scar may be quite visible. In women, this scar can typically be hidden by a bra strap or bikini. It is important to discuss the expected scar before surgery to clarify the patient's personal risks and rewards.

Designing markings before surgery is vital. Dermal lipectomies can usually be done with sedation and local anesthesia, but some patients require deep sedation or general anesthesia. The one- to two-hour outpatient operation is usually bilateral and may involve lifting the skin and fat layers to correct areas above and below. The incision is sutured in multiple layers over a surgical drain.

Drains are usually kept in place for five to seven days and sutures for one to two weeks. Mild to moderate bruising, tenderness, pain, and swelling are expected and may be severe for the first week after surgery. Returning to work and activity may be delayed between one and six weeks, depending on required activities. Rare complications include bleeding, infection, delayed healing of the incision, tissue necrosis, fluid buildup (seroma), and the disappointing results that are discussed under dermal lipectomies elsewhere in the book.

Chest-Wall Implants

Solid silicone chest-wall implants were originally developed to correct congenital deformities such as pectus excavatum. This deformity—in which the breastbone (sternum) is too deep in the chest, as well as other contour deformities of the ribs and chest—can be nicely corrected with these implants in both men and women. These implants can also be used in the chest wall for cosmetic augmentation, primarily in men who feel that the pectoralis major muscles are inadequately developed. Implant selection is critical because incorrect sizes will look unnatural.

Placement of chest-wall or pectoral implants is an outpatient procedure done under deep sedation or general anesthesia. Implants for congenital chest-wall deformities are usually placed through an incision in the upper abdomen near the lower tip of the breastbone or beneath the folds of the breasts. When augmenting the pectoral muscles in men, the incision is usually placed in the armpit to avoid visible scars on the chest wall. Chest-wall and pectoral implants should be placed in a pocket beneath the existing pectoralis major muscles, so the muscles will need to be lifted from the bone. After implant placement, the incision is sutured closed, typically without a drain. The incision is dressed circumferentially to minimize motion.

Pain after surgery may be significant but can be controlled with oral medication. Bruising and swelling occur but move down the torso with gravity and mostly resolve within several days. For several weeks, the residual swelling will make it appear as though the implants are too large. Before surgery, guidelines for resuming activity must be clear but may be modified, depending on progress after surgery. Daily activities must be restricted for seven to ten days, exercise and lifting must be avoided for three weeks, and more strenuous activity can usually be pursued after six weeks.

Although placing implants can improve chest contour, there are potential risks and complications. Bleeding could require reoperation for evacuation of old blood and control of any bleeding points. Infection can lead to significant problems, including the loss of the implant, so the patient should immediately report sign of infection and receive appropriate treatment. Signs include increasing pain, redness, or drainage from the incision. Treatment may include antibiotics, surgical drainage, or implant removal. If removed, waiting eight to twelve weeks is usually necessary before the implant can be replaced. Although unusual, the implant can cause an unacceptable level of discomfort, necessitating its removal. Fluid collections (seromas) increase the risk of infection and should be treated with aspiration, surgical drainage, or compression. Poor cosmetic results are possible and include improper size selection, displacement or rotation of the implant into a less ideal position, or having palpable or visible edges of the implant. As with any such problems with implants, any of these may require a revisional procedure.

Vaginal Rejuvenation

A woman may be dissatisfied with the appearance of her genitalia. This has become more common with the increasing incidence of genital hair removal and public exposure to nudity. The vulva consists of the clitoris, the vaginal canal (introitus), the outer folds (labia majora), and the inner folds (labia minora). The common cosmetic concerns are small labia majora, enlarged or elongated labia minora, or concealment of vagina by an excessive pubic region (mons pubis). These can be a source of significant embarrassment and discomfort for patients.

Labioplasty of the Outer Labia

Thin labia majora can cause the vulva to appear aged, the clitoris to appear phallic, or sexual enjoyment to decrease. Any of these concerns may prompt a person to seek treatment where the goal is to augment the labia majora. This can be done with fillers, but most surgeons prefer fat grafting (transferring fat from another part of the body) under anesthesia. All the fat grafts may not survive transplantation, but the cells that do survive can be permanent, and the surgery carries minimal risk. Bruising and discomfort may limit exercise and sexual activity for a week or two. Synthetic fillers are either temporary or run the risk of migration, clumping, or hardening with calcification, none of which are desired in this area. Recovery times are minimal, and sexual activity can usually be resumed within days.

Alternatively, an excessively large or full labia majora, either primarily or remnant after other body contouring surgeries, may need to be reduced. It is preferable to reduce with liposuction, but if there is too much skin present in this area, an excisional procedure may be necessary with several weeks healing time.

Labioplasty of the Inner Labia

The labia minora can become elongated, enlarged, or projecting. This can lead to embarrassment, avoidance of exposing oneself, poor hygiene, or discomfort either in routine activities or sexual activities. Through surgical treatment under local anesthesia with sedation, the excess tissue can be removed and closed with absorbable sutures in a way that does not interfere with sensation or function of the clitoris or the introitus. Six weeks of avoiding irritation, including intercourse, are needed to minimize the risks of both separating the incision and infection. Careful postoperative care and hygiene are necessary to help healing in this area. All sutures are absorbable.

Monsplasty

An excessively thick or long pubic region (mons pubis) can obscure the vulva, making hygiene, feminine care, and sexual intercourse difficult. Excess skin and fat are best addressed by removing these tissues by suspending up. This surgery is often incorporated into an abdominoplasty (tummy tuck) by thinning, lifting, and raising the mons pubis before closing the incision and then elevating the area. If an abdominoplasty is not planned, the skin and fat can be removed under local anesthesia, with or without sedation. The incision is usually hidden within or at the top of the pubic hair. Drains are usually not necessary, and absorbable sutures are frequently used. Significant exercise, sexual intercourse, and lifting should be avoided for six weeks after surgery.

Internal Vaginal Enhancement

With age and hormonal changes, the inner vagina can atrophy or stretch, compromising sexual satisfaction for one or both partners. This can be improved with either filling the soft tissues of the vagina, typically with fat grafting or laser tightening of the vagina. The former is truly adding back volume and requires sedation, and the latter is stimulating contraction with the same laser often used for tightening facial skin with wrinkles, carbon dioxide (CO_2), and is minimally painful, and return to normal activities is as soon as desired.

Scrotoplasty

Men may seek reduction in size or laxity of the scrotum. This relatively simple procedure involves resecting a portion of the scrotum and repairing it, typically with absorbable sutures. Postoperative support is beneficial.

Body Contouring of the Buttocks

The Buttocks

Most patients considering cosmetic surgery on the buttocks are concerned about excessive fat deposits that cause the buttocks to be excessively large, deflation, or progressive sagging that occurs with age. Some cases of fat excess may be solved by liposuction alone. Deflation or contour deficiency is typically noted in the upper buttock and can be corrected with silicone implants, fat injection, or autoaugmentation with elevated tissues. A sagging buttock can often be corrected by filling the upper buttocks (Brazilian buttock lift) but, when truly caused by excessive skin, may require a buttocks lift with skin and fat removal with placement and suspension in a better position.

Liposuction

The surgeon must carefully evaluate where fat is distributed on the buttock and how to correct it with liposuction. In general, the buttock excess is due to fat deposits in the lower midback (sacral diamond) on the upper part where each buttock meets the flank (hip rolls) and on the lower part where the buttock and thigh meet on each side (banana rolls). If there are indeed excessive fat deposits in these areas, the buttock can nicely be recontoured by removing these unwanted fat protrusions with the goal to help restore the loosely heart-shaped buttock. By thinning the sacral diamond, a definition between the two gluteal cheeks is defined. Reduction of the upper outer buttock helps separate the buttock from the flanks and abdomen. The banana roll, or gluteal fold area, which is the junction between the cheeks of the buttock and upper thigh, when poorly defined can often be corrected by liposuction of the upper portion of the thigh rather than of the buttock. Conservative liposuction may improve excessive fat in the cheek area, but aggressive liposuction of the cheeks can lead to significant sagging of the buttock, which can worsen a buttock deformity. Full buttock liposuction will often leave an undesired shape.

Buttock recontouring by liposuction is usually considered with the recontouring of the thighs and/or flanks. The advantages of recontouring the buttocks with liposuction are the tiny scars and easy recovery. The location of the scars will depend on the areas to be liposuctioned. The incisions may be placed at the junction of the buttock and thigh in the gluteal fold, in the flank area, or in the side of the thighs.

The Procedure

As discussed in its chapter, liposuction can be accomplished with wetting solution and intravenous sedation, or if this is part of a large liposuction or more invasive procedure, general anesthesia or epidural anesthesia may be necessary. It is usually done as an outpatient procedure without the need for observation overnight unless a large volume of fat is removed or other procedures are performed. Realistic goals must exist for liposuction because skin will not retract enough to match the removal of large amounts of diffuse fat from the buttock.

Gluteal Augmentation

Augmentation Using the Patient's Own Tissue

A deflated buttock can be corrected with a solid silicone implant, but most surgeons use fat injection or autoaugmentation by transplanting the patient's own tissue from a nearby area due to an improved safety profile. An aggressive change will likely require an implant. Fat injection is discussed in other chapters but involves fat transfer from the patient's own body. It is not possible to use donated fat. Fat is harvested with suction-assisted lipectomy and reinjected after preparation, usually in multiple planes in small aliquots throughout the existing fat and the gluteal muscles to augment the buttock. Large volumes are needed to create significant change, which increases risks of infection, asymmetry, and partial graft absorption. Staged fat grafting may be necessary for more significant change. The advantages of fat grafting is that there is no foreign body in the buttock with long-term potential for infection, migration, turning, or extrusion (exposure).

A patient with significant excess skin and subcutaneous tissue in the buttock or in the back or sides of the thighs is a good candidate for augmentation using a tissue transfer of a block of tissue from a nearby donor site on the patient's own body (autoaugmentation). This tissue can serve as an implant being elevated and rotated into position under the existing buttock skin after its epidermal layer of skin is removed. Standard surgical risks exist, but in addition, the transplanted tissue has reduced but intact blood supply, creating potential for necrosis, which can lead to either infection or gradual dissolution and disappearance. The procedure has a dual benefit in that it allows for removal of the excess skin and laxity while utilizing that tissue for a desired purpose. Recovery is similar to a buttock lift or body lift and requires compression, drains, and protection.

Augmentation Using Silicone Implants

A buttock implant made of solid silicone may be used to provide a shapelier or less saggy buttock. Injected (fluid) silicone has been used, but its use should be condemned because it tends to migrate and create granulomas, which can cause a long-term and disfiguring problem. It, unfortunately, is most often used in liquid form by nonmedical personnel attempting to achieve buttock enlargement without seeking appropriate medical care and is fraught with tremendous complications. Solid silicone implants may be placed in an outpatient setting and can generally be accomplished with local anesthesia and intravenous sedation, although some surgeons prefer general anesthesia or epidural anesthesia. The incision is most commonly made over the tailbone between the cheeks of the buttock. The implants are usually inserted beneath the fascia layer that surrounds the gluteus maximus, the large buttock muscle on each side. Placing the implant between the muscle and its fascia layer usually causes considerable discomfort or pain after surgery but less so than when placing in the muscle. Pain is readily controlled with prescribed medication. Placing the implant below the fascia also limits migration of the implant and reduces infection and extrusion risk, which are the major risks limiting the application of this technique.

Recovery

This is an inconvenient operation from which to recover. With any of these techniques, the buttock area will be bruised and swollen for several weeks, and again, bruising will descend to the thigh in time. Sitting and lying flat on the back are prohibited for one to two weeks after the operation. The patient must walk during early recovery to prevent serious complications such as venous thrombosis, but mobility must be tenuous and guarded. Positioning is best facedown or on sides or with significant padding to sit or sleep on one's back. Activities are slowly allowed over a few weeks with guidance from the surgeon. Major risks include bleeding, infection, prolonged pain, delayed healing, unsightly scars, or poor result caused by undercorrection, overcorrection, improper placement of the implant, or asymmetry in appearance. If there is bleeding at the site of surgery, it can require reoperation for evacuation of the hematoma and control of any bleeding.

Complications

A silicone implant can cause additional risks and complications. The most significant problem after placement of a foreign implant is infection, which first appears as increasing pain, redness, and drainage. Infection can lead to the loss of the implant and systemic infection, so immediate, appropriate management by the surgeon is critical.

The buttock area is exposed to minor trauma while walking, sleeping, sitting, and going about doing many other daily activities, so it is quite possible to disrupt the suture line and have an area of the incision separate. This is a minor problem if an implant is not exposed, and it can be corrected with local incision care. Implant migration can lead to deformity, asymmetry, or even implant extrusion if it protrudes through the incision, which would require implant removal.

It is not unusual to collect fluid in the pocket around the implant, called a seroma. Any significant collection of fluid may require aspiration by inserting a needle into the pocket and withdrawing the fluid. This may need to be repeated on several occasions, or a drain may need to be placed. A compression garment or pressure dressing that wraps the body can limit recurrence.

Although unusual, the implant can cause an unacceptable level of discomfort for a prolonged period because it may compress muscles or nerves. On occasion, this may necessitate implant removal.

The scars are designed to be well hidden under clothing or a bathing suit, but an abnormally overgrown (hypertrophic) scar may require treatment with cortisone injections and/or silicone pressure dressings. A poor cosmetic result can result from an improper selection of implant size, displacement, or rotation of the implant into a less ideal position, an asymmetric position, or having palpable or visible edges of the implant. Each of these will require surgical revision.

Buttock Dermal Lipectomy (Buttock Lift, or Fanny Tuck)

Buttock dermal lipectomy may be referred to as a buttock lift, or fanny tuck, and involves removing excess sagging skin and fat of the buttock area. The area to be surgically removed will be marked before surgery with the patient standing in an upright position The exact level on the buttock cheek where skin and fat are to be removed will be determined by the patient's individual shape, but it is almost always designed on the upper portion of the buttock, where a scar can be hidden by underwear or a bathing suit.

In most cases, surgeons avoid doing a direct excision in the gluteal fold because leg motion pulls on this location, making it more prone to wound-healing problems caused by tension. However, a scar in the gluteal fold can theoretically be hidden, and a smaller excision may be safely performed in this location. However, a larger excision may disrupt this natural crease and contour between the lower buttocks and thigh.

The Procedure

The operation may be done with intravenous sedation and local anesthesia, epidural anesthesia, or general anesthesia, depending on the amount of tissue to be removed, the surgeon's preference, and the patient's tolerance of lying flat on the stomach or on alternating sides during the procedure. Removal of skin and fat is performed meticulously. Lifting and moving some adjacent tissue may be necessary to reduce tension. After skin and fat are removed, the incision is closed with multiple layers of sutures. Suction drains are usually placed, and the incision is typically reinforced with dressings and a lower-body compression garment.

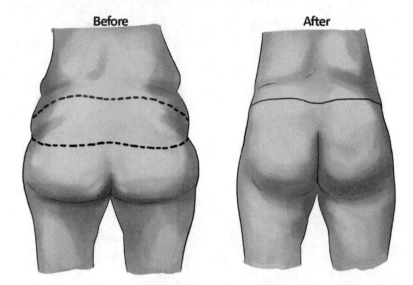

Figure 62. Buttock Lift

Recovery

After surgery, the buttock area will be sore and tender, requiring prescribed pain medication. The pain will begin to resolve in several days, but the discomfort can last for ten to fourteen days. Sitting and bending the hips place undue tension on the stitches and should be minimized for two weeks, as should lying on the back, which additionally stresses the healing incision by reducing blood flow to the area. Laying on the belly or sides is preferred. The stitches, if nonabsorbable, are removed between two and three weeks after surgery. Activity will be quite limited until the second to third week after surgery, and it will be four to six weeks before exercise can resume and most people are able to return to work.

Bruising is significant and will spread down the thighs with gravity but begins to resolve after several days. In most instances, bruising is gone within one to two weeks. The lower-body support garment is necessary for at least two weeks and may be recommended for longer, especially if the procedure is done in conjunction with liposuction.

BODY CONTOURING OF THE UPPER EXTREMITIES

The Arms

Dissatisfaction with the arms is frequently due to fat deposits in the upper part of the arm and armpit and/or to hanging, drooping skin in the upper arm. This is a common problem, even for individuals who are only slightly or moderately overweight. The deposit of fat in the upper arms causes an increase in arm circumference. As people age, gravity on the underportion of the arm results in a progressive sagging of the skin, which can be exacerbated by excess fat. In some instances, these excess tissues are noted even in young people, especially those who have lost weight either with diet, exercise, postpregnancy, or bypass surgery. The problem can be treated with liposuction or dermal lipectomy of the excess skin and fat or with some combination of these techniques.

Liposuction

Individuals with moderate fat deposition may be candidates for liposuction alone. The advantage of this operation is that the scars can be limited to small incisions in the armpit and/or elbow area, where they are not very visible. The fat is removed by liposuction, as discussed in its chapter. The amount of fat that can be removed aesthetically is limited by the ability of the skin to contract. If too much fat is removed or the skin is already lax and sagging, additional sag created by liposuction and deflation of the tissues can be equally or even more displeasing.

Liposuction of the arms can be accomplished with sedation and local anesthesia. After liposuction, the arm should be dressed with compression, either a garment or a wrap worn continuously until the skin has contracted down, typically two to four weeks. Significant pain occurs postoperatively but should resolve within five to seven days. Bruising should resolve within two weeks, whereas swelling will decrease slowly over a six-week period. As with all liposuctions, the swelling can obscure the final result for months.

Brachioplasty

Removal of excess skin or removal of excess skin and fat (dermal lipectomy) from the upper arm is known as a brachioplasty and is a common operation. Brachioplasty is indicated for excessive, hanging skin of the upper arms with minimal to moderate excess fat, as is commonly seen with significant weight loss. It is not recommended for generally obese patient with large upper arms because of a much greater complication rate. Mild to moderate amounts of loose skin can be expected to contract when treated with liposuction, but more significant laxity requires surgical removal of skin as well. Skin must be more lax than fat is excessive to minimize the tension on the stitches, which can reduce flow through the vessels or delay healing.

Surgical excision of skin and fat will result in scars on the arm, but these can be well tolerated and hidden when tension is minimized. If only a small amount of skin needs to be removed and pulled up toward the armpit, the excision can be performed across the armpit with suspension of the deep arm fascia to the fascia in the armpit, resulting in a final scar that is well hidden in the armpit crease. If circumferential excess skin extends down to the elbow, the skin excision may require a scar that extends longitudinally from the armpit to the elbow, a scar that can be quite visible when the arms are raised but is usually hidden in common positions with the elbows at the side. Many complex designs exist, and the excision is designed to leave a final scar on the inner aspect of the arm with a final scar that is as short as possible. The length of the scar is driven by the amount of excess skin removed. In certain patients, it is appropriate to combine this excision with the removal of excess chest or even breast tissue.

The Procedure

A brachioplasty is usually done as an outpatient procedure. The skin and fat to be removed will be marked before surgery with the patient in a sitting and standing position. The procedure is typically performed, with the patient lying in a supine (back) position with the arms out. In most cases, sedation with local or tumescent anesthesia is adequate, but general anesthesia may be necessary for certain patients. After the removal of excess skin and fat in the predesigned pattern, which may extend onto the chest, tension is minimized on stitches at the skin closure via good excision design and closure in layers, most notably suspension of the brachial (arm) muscle fascia to the axillary (armpit) fascia. Usually, stitches are placed under the skin to minimize scarring, and skin closure is reinforced with adhesive surgical tape and a compression dressing.

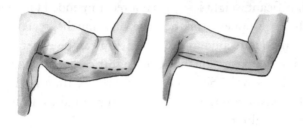

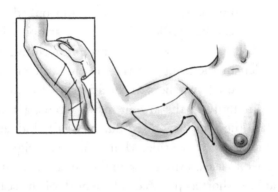

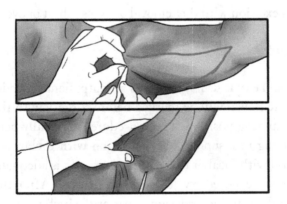

Figure 63. Brachioplasty / Arm Lift:
1. Ellipse 2. L-shaped with extension onto chest

Recovery

With any significant excision, suction drains are frequently used to reduce fluid and blood collections beneath the raised skin. The drains will be removed once drainage slows, usually one to seven days. A light, circumferential compression dressing is helpful in the first few weeks to limit swelling and healing problems. Stitches, if nonabsorbable, are usually removed by the third week after surgery. Moderate discomfort and pain requiring prescribed pain medication in the initial days after the procedure is expected but will slowly resolve over the first week or two. Most patients can return to work, dependent upon the expected activities, after one or two weeks, but exercise should be avoided for at least three weeks and then slowly resumed. Strenuous activities should be avoided for six weeks after the operation.

Complications

Complications are similar to those of other dermal lipectomies. A collection of fluid and/or blood beneath the skin flaps (seroma or hematoma) may require aspiration with a needle or surgical drain. If skin edges have impaired blood supply or drainage, delayed healing or actual skin slough may occur. Because the operation requires lifting the skin, there is a small risk of loss of skin at, and/or separation of, the incision edges. If this does occur, it will delay recuperation and will require treatment with dressing changes.

Many nerves are in the armpit and upper arm, so there is a slight risk of injury to sensory and motor nerves. If a sensory nerve is cut, bruised, or injured, numbness in the area served by the nerve will probably result. Because the arm skin has many sensory nerves, this is often not a major problem or even noticed. But in rare circumstances, it can lead to permanent numbness or an annoying or even painful sensation. Motor nerves are much less likely to be damaged because they travel more deeply and their paths are much more predictable, so problems moving the arm or hand are very unlikely.

Although most scars are narrow, flat, and fade in color, a widened, elevated, or discolored scar may result and may require treatment with cortisone injections and/or a pressure dressing with silicone. Swelling is expected after any surgery, but an unusual complication, called lymphedema, may lead to chronic (long-term) swelling of the arm if the incision is closed excessively tightly or a major disruption of lymph vessels occurs.

After any dermal lipectomy, the surgeon will leave extra skin at either end of the scar, estimating what will smooth out in time. Preventing it would require additional excision and lengthening of the scar at the first operation. If this "dog ear" does not smooth out, the scar still is shorter by removing this extra skin in a small, second procedure under local anesthesia after a couple months than if it were done at the first operation, so the final length of the scar is minimized.

The Forearms

The forearms can suffer from the same problems as the arms but usually to a far less significant degree. Excess fat can be liposuctioned but with caution due to the confluence of multiple nerves to the hands. Although extremely rare, excess skin can be excised either as a direct excision usually along the ulnar side or as an extension of the upper-arm brachioplasty.

The Hands

The hands are among the most heavily used and exposed parts of the body, and they typically show more age than any other. However, aging in the hands has received relatively little attention, aside from daily treatments such as moisturizers and creams that have limited effect. The changes that occur with age are related to sun exposure (causing wrinkles, altered pigmentation, and inelasticity), wind and chemical exposure (causing wrinkles and dry skin), and physiological tissue changes (causing skin excess and loss of fat under the skin). Most problems related to exposure are managed topically. Moisturizers and emollients can rehydrate the skin, but more aggressive, medical treatments are necessary for wrinkles, altered pigmentation, and inelasticity. These treatments include (1) skin resurfacing with chemical peels, dermabrasion, or lasers; (2) augmentation with fillers or fat grafting; and (3) direct excision of excess, lax skin.

Skin Resurfacing

Skin resurfacing with peels, dermabrasion, or lasers can be used on the hands to remove wrinkles, improve elasticity, remove areas of hyperpigmentation, and exfoliate the skin. However, conservative treatments are required as skin on the hands does not heal as readily as other skin because it has far fewer hair follicles and glands (appendages) from which deeply resurfaced skin grows and heals. This problem can lead to delayed healing, hypertrophic (overgrown) scarring, or hypopigmentation (lighter).

Fillers and Fat Grafting

The hands suffer from the loss of fat and muscle mass with age and begin to look thin and wrinkled, exacerbated by the visibility of tendons and veins. Numerous fillers have been attempted to augment the hand to create the youthful appearance of thick skin, but a thicker substance and larger volume is necessary to fill the relatively large area on the back of the hands enough to hide tendons and veins, so the more common fillers are Radiesse, Scultpra, Voluma, and fat. Grafting with fat taken from elsewhere on the body is the best option to return bulk to the skin of the thinning hand as there is not a volume limit and some of the fat injected is permanently present.

Fat can come from anywhere on the same patient's body but is typically taken from the abdomen, buttock, or thigh with a minimally invasive suction technique. The fat is prepared in one of many ways then deposited through multiple small incisions in layered passes below the skin of the hand in numerous small aliquots or deposit, being mindful of an even distribution.

The procedure can be done on an outpatient basis, but if both hands are treated, assistance with daily activities will be needed for a few days. A few small sutures can be removed at one week. Activities can be resumed during the first week, but swelling may be significant and can last for several weeks. Compression with gloves or tape can limit swelling after surgery.

Complications include infection, reabsorption of injected fat, uneven distribution of fat, injection of fat into a blood vessel or nerve. Some of the fat will be reabsorbed, but layered injection should result in an even texture, and retreatment should not be necessary. If uneven distribution occurs because of reabsorption or injection techniques, massage may even out the subcutaneous fat. If not, revision may be necessary with regrafting of more fat or redistribution with a cannula.

Infection and bleeding can lead to significant problems with any surgery, but these are uncommon with fat grafting. Even lower risk will be a fat embolus, which is very unlikely, especially in the hand, but can result in serious problems if a significant amount of fat travels to the lungs or brain. Injection into an artery can block blood flow and cause tissue loss on the hand. With the extensive knowledge of anatomy and safe techniques possessed by a well-trained plastic surgeon, the risks of injection into vessels and of nerve damage are very low.

Direct Excision

Direct excision can tighten the lax skin of the hands, and the scars can be made relatively inconspicuous. The excisions are usually performed along the side of the hand and fingers to minimize visibility of the scar on the palm or back of the hand. Precise anatomic knowledge is necessary in order to avoid damage to tendons, nerves, and vessels that are vital to the function of the hand, so a plastic surgeon with good credentials should be chosen. Sutures are typically removed at seven to ten days and recovery is usually rapid. Progression to normal activities by three to four weeks after surgery is typical.

Scars will result and may be functionally or cosmetically unacceptable if they are hypertrophic (ropy or overgrown) or contracted. Even with excision of excess skin, the hand may continue to appear aged because of thin skin and prominent veins and tendons, indicating a need for fillers or fat grafting.

Body Contouring of the Lower Extremities

The Thighs

Many patients, especially women, are unhappy with their thighs. The most common complaints are excessive fat, cellulite, or loose skin (see first image in Figure 64). A significant percentage of individuals seeking cosmetic surgery for large thighs are unhappy with excessive fat in the inner or outer thigh, which can be corrected with liposuction. Fat that encircles the thigh is more difficult to correct, as significant and circumferential fat reduction runs more risk of lax skin upon completion. Those individuals seeking correction of loose, hanging skin will require one of two procedures: thighplasty, an excision of skin and fat with lifting and moving of adjacent skin to lift the thigh, or dermal lipectomy, an excision of skin and fat.

Liposuction

Fat deposits in the thighs are notoriously difficult to lose even with strict diet and exercise programs. The most common area of concern is the "saddlebag" or "riding britches area" on the upper, outer portion of the thigh. Liposuction of this area can be done through an incision in the groin crease and from incisions in the lower abdomen and flank area.

Fat deposits on the insides of the thighs may be unsightly or uncomfortable as the thighs rub together when a person walks. This frequently treated area must be suctioned very carefully for several reasons. The inner thigh is full of important blood and lymph vessels and nerves that are at risk with liposuction in this area. Second, the inner-thigh skin is often thin and loose and does not recontour as well as the skin in the other parts of the thigh does. The inner thigh area can be suctioned through an incision in the groin crease toward the inside of the leg.

Fat in the rear, upper thigh, where the thigh and buttocks meet, can obliterate the normal gluteal folds in this location, making the buttock appear larger. Recontouring this "banana roll" with liposuction works well here, and it is usually done with an incision in the crease below the buttock.

For adiposity surrounding the whole thigh, the correction will be more difficult; however, the thigh can be suctioned circumferentially around the entire leg through multiple incisions to access and recontour large thighs. Several treatments may be necessary to remove the desired amount of fat safely, but even a series of surgeries is not without risk. As with any other liposuction, the major concerns are asymmetry, contour irregularities, seromas, incomplete correction, and excessive laxity due to deflation.

Thighplasty (Thigh Lift) and Thigh Dermal Lipectomy

Significant excess skin and thigh fat can be removed by excision. Both the thighplasty and a thigh dermal lipectomy procedures will remove fat, correct contour deformity, and improve the overall body contour, but these operations can cause visible scarring. There are many designs for placement of the incisions and the resulting scars, and the design chosen depends on the surgeon's preference, the patient's preference, and the distribution of fat and excess skin (see Figure 64).

Direct excision of fatty deposits and overlying skin can be performed, but the scars may be obvious. A horizontal crescent excision in the groin or over the hip may be used to lift the thigh without major fat excision; it may also be combined with liposuction. More generalized fat deposits of the thighs require a circumferential skin and fat excision, which will result in a scar around the entire circumference of the thigh. However, these incisions are kept high in the groin crease and extend toward the hipbone on the sides to keep them in a bikini-line distribution. The surgeon may also use a vertical skin excision on the inner or outer half of the thigh to remove localized fat deposits. The outer-thigh excision tends to heal better and with fewer complications than the inner thigh does, but it is quite visible. Therefore, most techniques use a vertical inner-thigh excision despite its being close to major blood and lymph vessels and nerves. Often a medial upper-thigh crescent is added to this procedure.

The Procedure

The smaller excisions to correct localized areas in either the inner or outer thigh can be done with sedation and local anesthesia. The more extensive lifts and dermal lipectomies generally require deep sedation, general anesthesia, or epidural block. The operation itself will take two to four hours, depending on the extent of the procedure planned and necessary liposuction. Smaller corrections may be done on an outpatient basis, but more extensive operations will require at least an overnight stay.

Possibly the most important step of the operation, the areas to be corrected and the skin incisions should be marked with the patient standing in an upright position before surgery begins. The thigh is lifted after removing excess tissue and loosening surrounding tissues as needed. Here is the next step: The tough system of fascia that runs throughout the outer (superficial) layers of the thigh must be suspended to a stable structure of the pelvis to reduce tension on the skin with heavy, typically permanent sutures. Precise closure of the skin and superficial layers further supports the elevation. Suction drains will be placed, and all incision lines will be sutured in multiple layers.

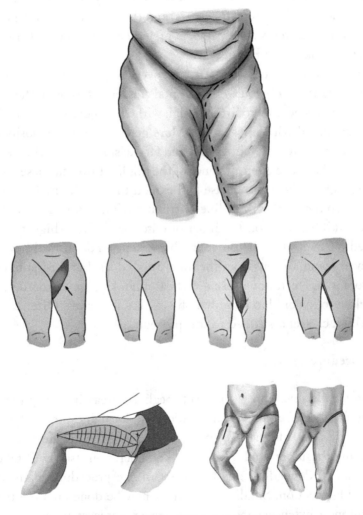

Figure 64. Thighplasty / Thigh Lift: 1. Preop laxity 2. Groin Crescent excision 3. L-shaped Thigh plasty 4. T-shaped Thigh Plasty 5. Lateral Thigh Lift

Recovery

Drains are removed when drainage slows, typically at one to two weeks. The thighs will be bruised, tender, and swollen. Symptoms may range from discomfort to significant pain. The pain should be manageable with prescribed pain medication. Stitches, if nonabsorbable, are removed at two to three weeks. Swelling should begin to resolve within a week or so, but it will be several weeks before the contour improvement can be appreciated and several months before the final contour is achieved. Return to work and activity depends on the extent of the surgery. With limited correction, it may be as short as a week, but more significant operations require longer periods of recuperation, typically two to three weeks before returning to work and four to six weeks before strenuous activity and exercise are resumed slowly.

Complications

Complications include bleeding, infection, delayed incision healing, tissue necrosis, seroma, and disappointing results, among other general surgical risks. Bleeding, while not common, can occur after any surgical procedure. Any significant collection of blood beneath the site of the operation can require another operation to evacuate the blood. Significant infection is rare, although superficial infections around the incision may occur, especially in the incisions in the groin crease as this area tends to be moist and easily macerated, and it is not unusual to have mild skin separation, drainage, and delayed healing; however, these should heal within a few weeks when treated with local cleansing and dressing changes. If there is a true infection, this healing process can require a surgical debridement or clean up and take much longer to heal.

Any time skin is lifted, it has a reduced blood supply that may be inadequate to keep a portion of skin alive. Rarely, portions of skin, especially those bearing the weight of the lift, will die and need to be either treated with dressing changes or, if severe enough, surgically removed.

Seromas may occur with any incision but are particularly troublesome in the inner thigh because of underlying lymph nodes and lymphatic vessels. If these are affected during the operation, fluids will accumulate under the incisions after the drains are removed. If a seroma is large enough, it may require aspiration by insertion of a needle and syringe or replacement of the drain.

Although most individuals are pleased with the aesthetic recontouring, these are difficult procedures, and there may be asymmetries between the two sides. A poor contour can be left behind if too much or too little tissue is removed. If too much tissue is removed from the inner thighs, it can pull on the vulva and labia, distorting the vaginal opening, but this is an unusual complication that can be corrected by reoperation. Removing a large amount of tissue between the lower buttocks and thigh may cause a loss of the natural junction between these two areas.

Many of these operations do lead to visible scarring, and the scars will remain red and noticeable in the early months. They will begin to fade and soften by the third month after surgery. The scars will fully mature by twelve to eighteen months. Any scars, but particularly the scars on the thin skin of the inner portion of the thighs, may widen. Thick, ropy scars and wide scars can be limited if a surgeon uses appropriate deep support, which reduces tension on the skin closure. It is important for the patient to understand the location and severity of scars before proceeding with a thigh lift or dermal lipectomy.

The Knees and Lower Leg

The knees and lower leg may also have skin or fat excess, leading someone to consult a plastic surgeon. Excess skin in this area is difficult to treat because of the high visibility of resulting scars and the number of important nerves and vessels traveling beneath the skin. Thus, dermal lipectomy (removal of excess skin and fat) is rarely appropriate, and we do not discuss it here. Excess fat of the knees or lower legs can be treated effectively with liposuction, but this procedure has higher risk, again because of the risks to vessels and nerves.

Not all patients are requesting a size or girth reduction of the lower legs: a growing number of men and some women are seeking augmentation of their calves.

Liposuction

Fat pockets on the insides of the knees are the most common complaint in the lower leg. This area responds well to liposuction and is commonly done at the same time as liposuction of the thighs and legs above the knee. An incision is usually made in the skin crease on the inside of the knee. If the knees are included in the liposuction, the postoperative compression garment should extend below the knees.

Only disproportionate, focal fat deposits below the knee should be removed with liposuction and—because the frequency of complications is higher—only by a surgeon who is well versed in the anatomy of blood vessels and nerves in the lower leg.

Excisional Procedure

Direct excision of fatty deposits and excess skin is possible on the lower leg but is exceedingly rare. If performed, this will be most likely on the inner upper calf, and care must be taken with the nerves to the foot. Even with meticulous surgery, the scars may be obvious.

Calf Implants

Individuals who are dissatisfied with the bulk of the lower portion of their legs may seek augmentation of the calf area with implants. The operation can be done with local anesthesia and sedation in an outpatient procedure but more commonly with general anesthesia. The implants are made of solid silicone and are typically inserted through incisions behind the knee and placed on top of the gastrocnemius (calf) muscles but under the fascia (muscle covering).

After the operation, the legs will be dressed with a circumferential, light-pressure dressing. The legs should be elevated as much as possible for three to four days with intermittent walking at least every two hours. It will be at least five to seven days before more normal activities can be resumed, and significant exercise will need to be postponed for at least six weeks. Pain is moderate and can be controlled with oral medication as it resolves for at least seven to ten days.

The most common problems after a calf implantation are dissatisfaction with the implant's appearance or discomfort resulting from its displacement.

Because the implant lies above the muscle, anything less than a perfectly shaped and sized implant may be noticeable.

Other complications include bleeding, infection, prolonged pain, seroma, implant migration, implant extrusion, injury to arteries or veins, nerve injury, or dysfunction of the muscle. If calf augmentation is strongly desired, a plastic surgeon experienced in calf augmentation should be chosen in order to reduce the significant risks of the operation.

COSMETIC SURGERY AFTER MASSIVE WEIGHT LOSS

Obesity is one of the major health crises today. The CDC reports that 1/3 (35% or 79 million) of Americans are overweight, 34% were obese, and 6% were morbidly obese. Weight-loss surgery, such as bariatric surgery, is the most effective long-term treatment for obesity, and over 100,000 procedures are performed annually. Massive weight-loss surgery and the need it creates for cosmetic surgery is a huge and rapidly expanding topic.

The American Society of Plastic Surgeons reports that its members— who include 94% of all board-certified plastic surgeons in the United States—performed 44,935 procedures for total body contouring after massive weight loss in 2014. The most common procedures include lower-body lift, abdominoplasty (tummy tuck), thigh lift, breast lift, and upper-arm lift (brachioplasty), which are all covered in detail in other chapters. To reduce the risk of these large surgeries, important considerations must be given to the evaluation before surgery, surgical planning and staging (timing), details to manage during surgery, and complications that may occur during surgery or recovery.

With most health insurance plans (but not all), these are cosmetic surgeries that are not covered by insurance. Combining certain procedures with reconstructive procedures (such as hernia repair) may allow for partial insurance coverage, but clear communication among the patient, the surgeon, and the insurance company is necessary to avoid confusion.

Early Consultation and Evaluation for Body Recontouring

In the evaluation before surgery, the surgeon and patient must discuss how massive weight loss occurred. In most cases, massive weight loss is the result of surgical treatment. However, if a patient experienced massive weight loss without weight-loss surgery, the cause requires further investigation. Although intentional massive weight loss is possible, other diseases (such as cancer or inflammatory bowel disease) must be ruled out. After determining the mechanism of weight loss, weight status and trends must be determined. Most of the weight is lost in the first year after weight-loss surgery, but every patient can be different. It is important for patients to have nearly achieved their goal weight and to have proven that they can maintain their current weight before proceeding with body recontouring surgery; rarely is this sooner than eighteen months after weight-loss surgery. If patients lose or gain significant weight in the future, the benefits of an otherwise successful plastic surgery are lost.

Several surgical options for weight loss are available. The major types of surgeries are to restrict the size of the stomach, to reduce the absorption of food and nutrients, and a combination of the two. Restrictive bariatric procedures are aimed at reducing the size of the stomach and therefore the amount of food eaten. This relatively simple procedure has a drawback: the remaining stomach has been shown to enlarge over time. Other bariatric procedures reduce the absorption of nutrients by bypassing portions of the gastrointestinal tract. The most common and most effective technique is a Roux-en-Y procedure, which reduces the size of the stomach and bypasses the portion of the small intestine that is closest to it.

Procedures that reduce absorption have significant relevance to body contouring. Because they can cause nutritional deficiencies and anemia, they can significantly impair healing after cosmetic elective procedures. Therefore, the surgeon will need a detailed history of each patient's medical conditions, surgical treatments, medications, and weight history. Laboratory blood tests can help assess a patient's nutritional status. Surgeons commonly order tests for protein levels in blood (albumin and prealbumin), blood counts (hemoglobin and hematocrit), clotting ability (coagulation times), electrolytes, and vitamin levels (A; B complex, including folate and B12; and C). Abnormal levels of any of these prompt further investigation.

Another important component of the preoperative evaluation is to determine the location of scars and potentially altered anatomy from any previous trauma, surgery, or individual traits that could alter standard options. Abdominal scars must also be examined for the possibility of a hernia that was caused by previous incisions.

Massive Weight-Loss Surgical Plan

After a thorough review of the history, physical exam, medical and nutritional status, and patient's goals, the surgical plan must be determined. Planning can often be complicated because many patients who experienced massive weight loss have numerous needs of varying severity. Skin laxity (loose skin) after significant weight loss is global—concerns often include facial laxity; eyelid bags (lid laxity and fat pouches); neck laxity; and drooping breasts, abdomen, buttocks, back, chest, thighs, arms, legs, or genitalia.

Certain procedures can be paired, and therefore, staging in the order of patient priorities can minimize the total number of operations needed while maintaining critical safety. Each operative plan is tailored to the patient, but common combinations include the following:

Stage 1 = Torso surgery (abdominoplasty or panniculectomy or lower-body lift)

Stage 2 = Breast surgery (lift and/or implants) and upper extremities (brachioplasty, hands)

Stage 3 = Facial aging (face, neck, brow, eyelids, mouth, and chin)

Stage 4 = Thighs and buttock and genitalia

The Procedures

The procedures are similar as to the primary chapters on each procedure, but typically, a greater amount of skin must be removed, which increases the risks of impaired cosmesis and healing. Also due to the global changes and skin laxity in patients, blending the procedures into the nonoperatively improved parts of the body is important. And while combinations may increase the risks of surgery, overall, it is safer for these patients to have a plan for surgeries that minimizes their trips to the operating room.

It is much more common to perform multiple stages as well as the more aggressive circumferential body lifts, staged thigh lifts, extended mastopexy, or brachioplasty to include the chest wall. This makes this population of patients more challenging.

General Concerns

The surgical details are similar to those outlined in other chapters, but certain additional considerations are vital. If a patient has a hernia that was caused by previous incisions or that lies in the abdominal muscles, repairing the hernia can be combined with the body contouring stage, but this does increase the risks of the operation. As discussed above, adequate nutritional status is mandatory to maximize the healing ability of the large incisions needed in these elective procedures, in which large amounts of skin must be removed and redraped. Layers of soft tissue that are stronger and deeper than skin must be sutured and suspended higher—this is pivotal to maximizing lift and minimizing scars in these procedures. Most areas have well-defined structures called fascia around the muscles that can be lifted and secured with sutures during surgery.

Due to the large size of the areas treated and the potential for malnutrition in patients who have achieved massive weight loss, pockets or collections of fluid or blood that the body is not able to clear (seromas or hematomas) are more likely to occur than in other patients undergoing cosmetic surgery. Therefore, aggressively draining and compressing these collections are important to minimize complications after surgery caused by infections that result when these pockets occur. Both drainage and compression may be necessary for longer periods of time than in most patients to improve healing after massive weight-loss surgery, so drains are used for three to six weeks, and compression is applied for two to four months.

Risk factors to control during surgery and recovery can be minimized by thoroughly investigating major medical risks ahead of time—these are diabetes, heart attack, anemia, blood clots in the legs or lungs (deep vein thrombosis or pulmonary embolus), and organ failure. Aggressive preventive treatment against blood clots is recommended by the American Society of Plastic Surgeons and may require the injection of blood thinners at home before and/or after surgery.

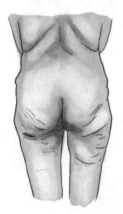 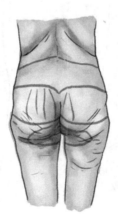 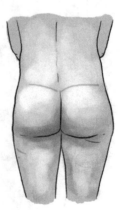

Figure 65: 1. Preop laxity of posterior after massive weight loss. 2. Markings. 3. Postop

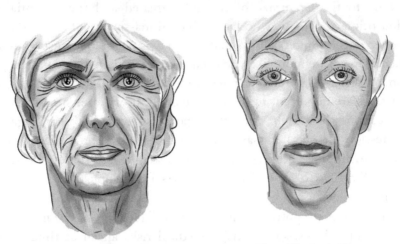

Figure 66: 1. Preop laxity of Brow, eyes, Face, Neck. 2. Postop

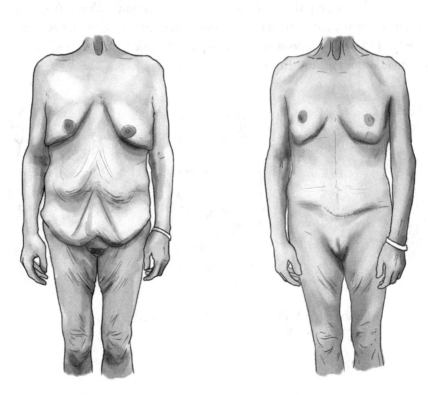

**Figure 67: 1. Preop laxity of Chest, Breasts, Abdomen,
Genitalia, Arms, and Thighs. 2. Postop**

COSMETIC SURGERY IN MEN

The techniques used for cosmetic surgery are similar in men and women, but there are several problems unique to men as well as anatomic and lifestyle preferences that require modification of surgical procedures. These differences are noted here and should be incorporated with additional information in the appropriate chapters. According to statistics from the American Society of Plastic Surgeons, approximately 15% of cosmetic procedures are performed in men and total volume has nearly doubled since 1992. The most common procedure remains rhinoplasty, but other common operations include eyelid surgery, liposuction, hair transplantation, and gynecomastia correction. During that same era, the incidence of male liposuction has tripled, while male face-lift has doubled.

The Skin

Male facial skin tends to be thicker and more vascular than that of a female, mostly as a result of hair follicles and skin appendages in the beard region of the face. Men also have a greater percentage of body water than do women and a significant difference in circulating hormones, which affect skin aging in an unclear way. The anatomy, age, and environmentally related changes and treatment options are the same as those outlined in the chapter on facial rejuvenation, but there are special male considerations. Skin-care products are essentially developed and marketed for women, including the packaging, marketing, colors, and fragrances. Men are less conditioned to the use of routine products but can benefit just as much from preventive care, including sunscreen, moisturizers, exfoliants, and other products discussed in the chapter on skin.

Rhinophyma

Rhinophyma is the end stage of a severe acne rosacea with overgrowth of the sebaceous glands of the nasal skin, characterized by a red, thickened and bulbous nose. Correction can be done as an outpatient procedure under local anesthesia, possibly with oral or intravenous sedation. The abnormal skin can be removed by a number of techniques including dermabrasion, CO_2 or erbium resurfacing laser, or excision with an electrically heated knife. The abnormal tissues are removed, but the deeper skin structures remain, allowing for epithelization, healing via the growth of new skin from deep appendages and dermis. After surgery, the nose is dressed with antibiotic ointment or a moist, nonstick dressing that requires changing at least daily with soap and water cleansing to limit crusting. Most of the wound will heal within seven to ten days, although additional scattered areas may take another four to five days. Erythema should subside within a month, but low-grade redness may persist due to persistent acne rosacea, which can be managed with topicals and oral antibiotics.

Minimally Invasive Procedures

Men often desire improvement in the appearance of acne scars, altered pigmentation, and facial wrinkles and can benefit from chemical peels, dermabrasion, and resurfacing laser. The preoperative and intraoperative considerations are universal, but the postoperative care is more complicated in men. Once their skin heals in seven to ten days after the procedure, the skin of males and females alike is erythematous (pink or red) for up to several months with the CO2 laser or deep peels. Women can use makeup to camouflage the redness, but most men are reluctant to use cosmetics. For this reason, a series of light peels, a superficial medium peel, or a superficial laser resurfacing with an Erbium:YAG may be more appropriate for those not prepared to use makeup since the erythema is less severe and shorter lasting. Despite a massive proportion of female usage, the treatment modalities for the correction and improvement of fine wrinkles and contour depressions with Botox, fillers, and fat grafting are equally effective in men and women, as discussed in detail elsewhere. Similarly, spider veins, although more common in women, do occur in men and are also amenable to electrodesiccation, sclerosis, and laser treatments.

Hair and Hair Loss

Half of all men will notice obvious hair loss by the fifth decade and close to 70% loss at some point during their lifetime. The peak incidence is between twenty and fifty, although some individuals experience hair thinning soon after the onset of puberty. Hair loss is the number 1 cosmetic concern for which men seek counsel. It can cause an inordinate degree of social discomfort and anxiety, especially in younger individuals. Even in the most resilient man, hair loss is a reminder of the relentless indignities of the aging process. There are a number of potential causes for hair loss, but the overwhelming cause is male-pattern baldness, and the pathophysiology, as well as the treatment of hair loss, is discussed in its own chapter.

Facial Rejuvenation

Facial rejuvenation is rapidly gaining acceptance among males, and its incidence is rapidly expanding. Although most men seeking facial rejuvenation are middle-aged professionals between fifty and sixty, it is certainly not limited to this age group. The techniques for male facial rejuvenation are similar to those discussed elsewhere, but there are important features in men that will affect the surgical technique. In a face-lift, the adjusted position of hair-bearing skin must be taken into consideration as it is excised. This will adjust the beard distribution, and if the incision is behind the tragus (cartilaginous prominence in front of the ear), as is often done in women, hair-bearing skin will be moved inside the ear, compromising cosmesis, hygiene, and shaving. The effect on the sideburn location must also be considered. Excision in the scalp adjusts and sometimes eliminates the sideburn, a desired feature in men as opposed to women. Similarly, many men have less hair-bearing scalp behind the ear, and an excision in the hairline, as is common in women, can alter the posterior hairline and leave a large step-off. Therefore, the face-lift incision is usually placed in front of the ear and along the existing sideburn, temple hairline, and posterior hairline. Most scars heal imperceptibly, but if a poor scar results, it is usually visible since there is no longer hair surrounding the scar on both sides. Also, the hair-bearing (bearded) facial skin is thicker and more vascular, requiring tedious hemostasis (control of bleeding) in order to curb the increased risk of bleeding complications such as hematoma.

Neck

Male neck complaints are usually the excess skin and fat beneath the chin and of absence of a sharp cervico-mandibular angle between the neck and the face, which in youth is ideally near 90°. If part of the problem is a retruded or deficient chin, a chin augmentation either with an implant or chin advancement may suffice. Usually, however, there is an excess tissue in the submental region due to gravity, skin laxity, and excess fat. If the problem is due to excess fat with minimal skin laxity, the fat can be removed by suction lipectomy, and some skin contraction will occur. If there is significant excess skin or skin with poor tone, skin excision is necessary. A small amount of excess skin can be removed with a transverse excision that can be well hidden beneath the chin. Larger amounts of skin, however, are most commonly removed with a traditional face-lift. If a full face-lift is not desired, the excess skin can be removed with a horizontal and vertical excision of the skin, typically with Z-plasty (interdigitation of tissue flaps to disrupt the scar lines and adjust angles of tension) along the mid neck. The scar is usually acceptable but can be quite large, extending from below the jaw to the thyroid cartilage (Adam's apple), and with poor healing scar, a noticeable scar could result.

Eyebrow/Forehead

The ideal male eyebrow is less arched and lies lower than the female brow, at or slightly above the supraorbital bony rim. The eyebrows can descend over the bony rim onto the upper lid, compromising vision or cosmesis, and elevation of the eyebrow can be an important component of upper-eyelid correction. The techniques for eyebrow and forehead lift are well described in their own chapter, but in males, the approach must be carefully correlated with the current and anticipated hairline and hair thickness. With thick hair, all approaches are acceptable, but transcoronal and endoscopic approaches are the most common. With a receding hairline, the incisions must be placed far back in the scalp to avoid a visible scar, and an endoscopic forehead lift can limit this risk. In patients with minimal hair, direct excision in a wrinkle or above the eyebrows is potentially less visible. As with any cosmetic surgery, the anticipated outcome, potential scars and risks, and reasons for technique selection should be discussed preoperatively.

Eyelids

Men tend to be less concerned than women about wrinkles in the eyelid skin than do women, but often seek blepharoplasty consultation for bags in the lower lids and excess sagging skin with or without protruding fat pads of the upper lids. More often than in women, there may be sufficient overhanging upper-eyelid skin or brow descent to obstruct peripheral vision. If a visual study can document obstruction of peripheral vision, upper-lid blepharoplasty and/or brow lift may be considered a reconstructive procedure covered by insurance.

The Nose

Men often seek rhinoplasty to correct an undesired size or shape of the nose or a crooked nose resulting from previous trauma. The crooked nose is usually due at least partially to a deviated septum, and if present, a septum deviated by trauma may obstruct airflow, which is a functional problem and may be covered by insurance. Men tend to have larger and stronger bone structure and facial features than women, and since the nose must relate to the rest of the face, rhinoplasty should be more conservative than in women in most instances. Potential difficulties include excessive reduction of the nasal tip or dorsum, resulting in a feminine nose that does not harmonize with the rest of the face. The thicker male nasal skin limits the ability to refine the nasal tip, and excessive sculpting of tip cartilages in an attempt to overcome thickened skin leads to loss of tip definition. Patients and surgeons must be aware that the cosmetic goals of a rhinoplasty are quite different for the two sexes, and desires to feminize the male nose must be extensively explored before proceeding.

The Ears

Men may be more self-conscious about prominent or protruding ears due to shorter hairstyles and less ability to camouflage ear abnormalities. An otoplasty, however, is technically the identical between the two sexes and is discussed in its own chapter.

The Chin and Jaws

An excessively prominent chin can be corrected with a reduction genioplasty, and a receding chin can be corrected with a chin implant or chin advancement. The general technique is similar between the sexes, but techniques or implants can be modified to enhance or maintain a stronger, more square chin than the more feminine pointed chin. Surgery may be delayed or avoided in patients who grow a beard to camouflage a prominent or weak chin.

Body Contour of the Torso and Extremities

With the rapid growth in cosmetic surgery, more males are seeking body contouring. As men age and put on weight, they tend to deposit fat in the lower abdomen around the waist (love handles, beer belly, or spare tire), thighs, back, and arms. These areas can be addressed with liposuction or excisional techniques. The flanks of men (love handles), thighs, back, and arms can usually be corrected with liposuction through small incision in creases or folds. In the male abdomen, excess fat is usually addressed with liposuction, but significant skin access requires similar excisional techniques: mini abdominoplasty, abdominoplasty, panniculectomy, or circumferential body lift. Technical details are modified to maintain the masculine body shape of narrow hips relative to shoulders. Preoperatively, it is important to determine the distribution of fat. Many male patients have central obesity due to fat on and around the bowel, which is obviously not correctable. Cellulite is less common in males. Some men in excellent shape have fat deposition in the abdomen, obscuring the muscular definition of the rectus muscle. Those seeking a six-pack appearance may be candidates for abdominal sculpting, liposuction of the subcutaneous fat overlying the muscles.

Although less common in men, the details of extremity procedures are similar between the two sexes, including brachioplasty (arm lift), thighplasty, calf implants, and hand rejuvenation. Scrotoplasties are an option for those men that feel that they have an elongated or stretched scrotum.

Liposuction techniques can be performed on an outpatient basis with sedation and local/tumescent anesthesia. Excisional procedures usually require deeper sedation or general anesthetic. Ultrasonic, laser, or power-assisted liposuction is more often beneficial in males due to the higher frequency of dense fat deposits. Recovery is similar to women, with moderate pain requiring prescribed narcotic medication for several days, an abdominal binder for ten days to three weeks, return to light duty in several days, exercise at three weeks, strenuous activities at four to six weeks, and bruising/swelling for several weeks.

The Chest and Breasts

Males have breasts but they are much simpler, nonfunctional organs in men. The cosmetic concerns are mainly limited to polythelia (accessory nipples), gynecomastia (male breast enlargement), and chest implants, as discussed previously. Accessory nipples can be observed or excised. Gynecomastia in youth is typically hormonal stimulation of glandular tissue, whereas in older men, it is usually due to fat deposition. Either deformity is amenable to suction lipectomy, but gland/breast bud excisional techniques are often combined in younger patients with gynecomastia. Severe deformities will require removal of skin and fat. Chest-wall implants can correct insufficient pectoralis muscle bulk and pectus deformities.

Conclusion

As one would expect, the surgeries between the two sexes are similar, but modifications must be made to maximize the aesthetics of surgical outcomes in a man versus a woman.

COSMETIC SURGERY IN ETHNIC GROUPS: SPECIAL CONSIDERATIONS

There has been a dramatic increase in the number of Hispanic, Asian, and African American patients seeking cosmetic surgery in the past decade. Statistics from the American Society of Plastic Surgeons indicate that in 2012, 11% of patients were Hispanic, 8% were African American, and 7% were Asian. The normal facial features for each of these groups are distinct, and each group has its own ideals of beauty. When choosing a doctor, every patient should know that a plastic surgeon must understand and respect these differences when evaluating an ethnic patient. Many cosmetic procedure essentials are the same for all races, but it is vital that the patient feels comfortable that the surgeon is able to refine surgical techniques to adjust for ethnic anatomic features and aging differences. The operative experience, anesthesia, and recovery after surgery are similar for all ethnic groups and are discussed in other chapters.

Aesthetic Surgery in African Americans

Important ethnic differences must be respected when considering surgical procedures. Because African Americans are prone to two different types of thick scars, existing scars can be the reason that a patient consults a plastic surgeon but must also be given extreme attention in planning elective, cosmetic procedures. African Americans' propensity for pigmentation changes after surgery must also be considered.

The most common reasons for cosmetic consultation in African Americans are abdominoplasty, scar modification, rhinoplasty, liposuction, and breast augmentation. Specific details in abdominoplasty, liposuction, and breast augmentation do not differ significantly among races, but facial and nasal characteristics are quite different in African American patients. The variations in anatomy and their effects on the desired results after surgery must be understood to avoid disappointing results.

Hypertrophic Scars and Keloids

African Americans are more prone to hypertrophic scars and keloids, and a personal or family history of either is pivotal in deciding to undergo cosmetic surgery because their formation can lead to disfiguration that is far beyond the potential benefits of cosmetic surgery. Both types form thick scars, but keloids extend beyond the original incision or wound into nearby skin and soft tissue; hypertrophic scars do not extend themselves in this way. The areas most prone to hypertrophic scars and keloids are the sternum (breastbone), arms, and ears, but any part of the body may be involved. Fortunately, the most visible parts of the body, the face, neck, and hands are less likely to suffer from these problems.

The best approach to hypertrophic scars and keloids is prevention or early intervention because they can be difficult to control. Any signs of scar hypertrophy should be treated with steroid injections with cortisone or triamcinolone) into the abnormal scar and silicone patch therapy. The cortisone injections can be repeated monthly for several months, but there is some risk of temporary or permanent light pigmentation because steroids are toxic to the cells that produce skin pigment. If silicone patch therapy does not soften or flatten the scar, a pressure garment can be initiated. Other adjuncts include laser therapy if persistent and radiation therapy if severe.

Established hypertrophic scars and large keloids often need to be surgically removed and reclosed with a minimally traumatic technique; this is followed by prophylactic immediate steroid injections and pressure therapy. In the case of an earlobe keloid, which can be seen after piercing, a specialized compression earring can provide the needed pressure after excision. Wearing this earring may be required for up to six months. Skin grafts can be used to cover areas that had large keloids or persistent keloids. In this situation, keloids usually do not form in the area of graft, but they can recur at the junction between the graft and native skin, which can result in an unattractive ring of keloid surrounding the graft.

Patients with recurrent keloids that have been treated appropriately with steroids, skin grafts, and pressure therapy may be candidates for excision, closure, and treatment with low-dose radiation after the procedure. The dose is typically 600 rem divided over three daily treatments; this is approximately one-tenth of the dose used to treat common, cancerous tumors. Although radiation is effective and its dosage is very low, its collective side effects over a lifetime should not be taken lightly—these include the promotion of cancers and, especially, sarcomas. Keloids and hypertrophic scars usually recur in the first few months; after six months, the future development of either is unlikely.

Skin Pigmentation Changes

African American skin is much more likely to develop abnormal pigment and discoloration after surgical manipulation. Possibilities are either hyperpigmentation (increased pigment, or darker color) or hypopigmentation (decreased pigment, or lighter color). In most patients, this does not preclude surgical care, but risks are high with topical treatments of fine wrinkles or acne scars with dermabrasion, chemical peels, or laser resurfacing. If such treatments are planned, a patch of skin, typically behind the ear, should be tested before the entire face is treated to determine a patient's susceptibility to such difficulties. If hyper- or hypopigmentation does occur, skin color will usually return to normal after two to three months or, in many instances, up to twelve to eighteen months. Hyperpigmentation may be reduced with routine use of a bleaching agent containing hydroquinone, while areas of hypopigmentation can only be covered with cosmetics once the incisions have completely restored normal skin (usually within a week after the procedure).

Aging

African American facial skin ages less dramatically than white skin does. Skin laxity and wrinkles, especially in the forehead, the eyelids, the crow's feet, and around the lips tend to be much less of a problem. However, in time, the facial soft tissues of all races suffer the effects of gravity and skin laxity. The most noticeable change is often in the midface, where the fatty tissue overlying the cheekbones descends, deepening the fold between the upper lip and cheek.

Correction of the midface is usually done in conjunction with a face-lift operation or lower-lid surgery (blepharoplasty). Incisions similar to those discussed elsewhere are used, and the scar in front of the ear is rarely complicated by hypertrophic or keloid scar formation. However, the scar behind the ear and into the hairline is prone to excessive scarring, so the severity of facial aging must be sufficient to justify this risk. Despite their risk of causing hypopigmentation, steroid injections should be initiated at the first sign of abnormal scarring.

Neck laxity can be addressed with a lower face-lift, with liposuction, or with direct removal of skin. Incisions in the thin neck skin do not tend to form excessive scarring or pigment changes, and liposuction further minimizes the chances of ill scarring because they require a lesser amount of skin excision and create smaller scars.

In all races, aging around the eyes shows itself as an increasing loosening and growth of extra skin, as well as the protrusion of fat pads, causing the appearance of bags; these are corrected by standard methods, as discussed in the section "Eyelids." Because brow sagging is much less common in African Americans than in whites, most African Americans will not require a brow lift, but occasionally, consideration may need to be given to a brow lift. If the changes in the lower eyelid are due primarily to fat protrusion and bags, an incision on the inside of the eyelid both allows for correction of fat compartments and avoids the need for a skin incision. Conversely, significant skin laxity in the lower eyelid requires removal of both excessive skin and fat through a standard blepharoplasty. Hypertrophic scarring and keloid formation are exceedingly unusual in the eyelids, but on occasion, the scar line will hyperpigment. Because of its proximity to the lash line, even a dark scar is usually well hidden, and the color tends to correct in time.

The Lips

A common complaint among African Americans presenting for cosmetic surgery is excessive fullness of the lips, which can be corrected after the desired amount of change is clear. The operation can be done either in a doctor's office or in an outpatient operating facility. With or without sedation, local anesthesia can be used to numb the lips and block the nerves in the lower lip and upper lip. For a limited correction, a horizontal ellipse of tissue is removed from inside the lip. In fuller lips, both a horizontal ellipse and a V-shaped wedge are excised to remove additional tissue, but the scars are still not visible because they are inside the lip. The incisions are closed with absorbable sutures that last for ten to fourteen days.

After surgery, the lip will be swollen and temporarily larger than before reduction, especially without strict adherence to frequent icing and elevating the head for the first twenty-four to forty-eight hours. Swelling will begin to resolve within ten to fourteen days, but complete resolution may take one to three months. Because it is easy to distort the lip by taking away too much tissue—and easy to reduce the lip farther by excising more mucosa at a second setting—removing less tissue is the norm at the initial procedure. As with any operation, other complications, such as bleeding, infection, or nerve injury are possible but are quite unusual events. Management could require antibiotics or reoperation to drain a hematoma. An injury to the nerve in the chin is rare and is usually due to an anesthetic injection rather than surgical trauma; it should resolve over weeks to months.

The Nose

Certain features characterize the African American nose, including a nose that is flatter, shorter, and wider than the white nose with wide flaring of the nostrils, which are oval in shape. At the consultation, the desired changes to the nasal features—as well as features the patient wishes to keep—must be discussed. While many patients seek a refinement of the nasal appearance while retaining its basic ethnic characteristics, others desire a completely different nasal appearance with loss of ethnic features and a more white appearance. In either case, it is imperative to maintain harmony between the nose and other facial structures. Although the specific techniques are similar to those used in a standard rhinoplasty, the patient must choose a plastic surgeon who is experienced in cosmetic surgery of the African American nose and who understands the patient's desires and concerns.

The nasal dorsum (roof of the nose) is often flat, short, and broad. Reshaping the dorsum requires augmentation of the nose, building it up with cartilage (from the septum of the nose or from the rib) or bone (from either the outer layer of the skull or pelvis). Cartilage from the septum is the most common graft because it is in the area already undergoing surgery, is easy to obtain, does not add significant time to the operation (especially when surgery on the septum is already planned), and does not require general anesthesia; however, the amount of graft is limited. While most rhinoplasties can be done under local anesthesia and sedation, remote grafts (from the skull, rib, or pelvis) usually require general anesthesia.

Significant nasal tip work usually requires opening the nose through an incision inside the nose and across the skin bridge between the nostrils. This is referred to as an open rhinoplasty, which gives the surgeon better visibility and allows the surgeon to work under the best conditions. It generally heals with an imperceptible scar. Definition and improved projection of the nasal tip can be achieved with the creative use of sutures or with cartilage grafts from the nasal septum, the ears, or both. Ear cartilage is soft and pliable and can be more precisely molded to augment the nasal tip. It can be obtained under local anesthesia through an incision behind the ear, leaving no obvious scar or ear deformity.

Flared nostrils can be modified by releasing the cartilage from the facial skeleton or by removing skin in the nostril floor or where the nostril meets the cheek. The potential problems with removing skin here can be airway and breathing problems, asymmetry of the nose, or poor appearance of scars. Thorough evaluation before surgery and precise surgical technique can prevent breathing problems and asymmetry, and the resulting scars are occasionally poor but are usually imperceptible. More details about this surgery and its recovery are discussed in its chapter.

Aesthetic Surgery in Asian Patients

As in all groups, the demand for cosmetic surgery has increased in the Asian population. The most common cosmetic surgeries in the Asian population are rhinoplasty (nose reshaping), breast augmentation, and eyelid surgery. Many cosmetic procedures such as body contouring (liposuction, breast surgery, and abdominoplasty) and facial rejuvenation (face-lift, brow lift, and chin surgery) are essentially the same as the procedures discussed in other chapters, but two areas that require special attention in Asian patients are the eyelids and the nose. Most Asians seeking cosmetic procedures of the eyelid and nose are not looking to westernize their features, as has been suggested by some. Rather, they seek a change in a facial feature to satisfy their sense of aesthetics and beauty.

Asian Upper Eyelids

Cosmetic blepharoplasty (eyelid reshaping) is often sought by Asians whose upper eyelids have a web or fold of skin at the inner aspect of the eyelid adjacent to the nose or who do not have a supratarsal or a palpebral crease. The inner epicanthal fold is also known as a Mongolian fold (see Figure 68).

In eyes with a poorly defined supratarsal crease, there is no, or a very low, attachment between the eyelid skin and the levator muscle that opens the eyelid. As a result, the eyelid appears to have no fold and to be full because fat migrates downward, under the eyelid skin. The surgical procedure is directed at correcting the inner upper eyelid web and creating a well-defined supratarsal fold (see Figure 68). The supratarsal fold is readily seen in white eyelids, but it is also seen in many Asian eyes; therefore, when done correctly, creating the fold and suspending the periorbital fat can change the eyelids without making the patient appear Western.

The Asian upper blepharoplasty is often referred to as the double-eyelid operation, and it can be done under local anesthesia in an outpatient setting. Two techniques are available: (1) using an incision to remove excess skin and fat from the upper eyelid before recreating the supratarsal fold or (2) using quilting sutures without an incision. In either case, a row of stitches is designed to attach the skin to the underlying levator muscle that is normally present. Using the first technique—with an incision—allows the surgeon to remove excess fat in the superficial eyelid to more securely fix the skin to the levator muscle. The quilting technique, which is more common in Asia and is not widely performed in the United States, tends to be less predictable and less durable than with the incision technique.

The web on the inner aspect of the eyelid can be corrected with local tissue rearrangement. Caution is advised because correction of this web can result in a noticeable or hypertrophic scar. Although scarring is unlikely, the risk is higher in patients with pigmented skin, as previously discussed.

ASIAN

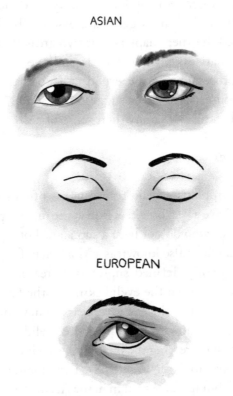

EUROPEAN

Figure 68: Asian eyes 1. Examples 2. Westernization of Asian Eyes 3. Aged European eyes

Asian Nose

There is a great deal of variability in the appearance of the nose among different Asian ethnic groups, but the typical Asian nose is characterized by a flat nasal dorsum (top of the nose), a relative lack of projection of the nasal tip, and thicker nasal skin than is seen in whites. The most common reason that patients consult cosmetic surgeons is the flat, underprojecting nose. In planning, surgeons must elicit the patient's desired amount of modification and must determine how to maintain harmony between the nose and other facial features. A thin, projecting nose will not balance a wide, flat face, just as a wide, flat nose will not balance a long, thin face.

The operation can be performed under local or general anesthesia in an outpatient setting either through incisions inside the nose or by opening the nose with a technique that includes an incision across the skin that bridges the nostrils. The basic operative approaches are described in its chapter, but an emphasis is placed on thinning the soft tissues of the nose, strengthening the nasal tip, and augmenting the nasal dorsum. While the skin itself should not be removed or thinned, removing fibrous, fatty tissue from the bone and cartilage underneath effectively reduces the apparent thickness of the skin and soft tissues. Nasal tip projection can be achieved with a combination of sculpting the nasal cartilages and adding cartilage grafts taken from the nasal septum or the ear.

Augmentation of the nasal dorsum is the major portion of the procedure. It can be done either with grafts of the patient's own cartilage or bone or with synthetic materials. Minor dorsal augmentation can be obtained with a cartilage graft from the nasal septum or ear, which can be readily obtained during the rhinoplasty procedure with little added operating time or expense. Major augmentation requires rib cartilage, rib bone, a bioprosthetic material, or synthetic implants. Using rib cartilage or bone obviously requires a major additional surgical site and general anesthesia. Large pieces of rib cartilage are prone to warping and may require internal fixation with a wire during healing. Bone is obviously not likely to change shape, but it is unforgiving and can be difficult to mold to the desired shape. If, however, previous augmentation has failed because the cartilage has warped or synthetic implants have became infected or moved out of position, bone graft augmentation may be the best option. Donor sites for bone include the pelvis and the outer layer of the skull, as discussed in the chapter on nose.

Synthetic implants, especially silicone, are commonly used in Asia, and the advantage of using these is that no procedure is required to obtain donor cartilage or bone. This greatly simplifies the operation and reduces recovery, but the risk of complications after surgery is greater with the use of synthetic materials (infection, exposure, and extrusion), as discussed in the minimally invasive chapter.

Bioprosthetic materials are products that are manufactured from human or animal tissue for use in various ways, including nasal augmentation. Their risks are a hybrid of the above two (using the patient's own donor tissue versus using synthetic implants). Using bioprostheses carries increased risk of infection, migration, extrusion, and absorption than using a patient's own tissue does, but risks are lower than with synthetic implants because these materials are less foreign to the body. The products are usually harvested from skin, mucous membranes, cartilage, or bone. They are then treated in a variety of ways to reduce the risk of the spread of disease, but patients must agree to use such a product before this option is selected.

Aesthetic Surgery in Hispanic Patients

The cosmetic procedures selected by Hispanic patients are in line with the cosmetic procedures desired by the general population. The most common procedures are breast augmentation, liposuction, and rhinoplasty (nose reshaping). While the details and techniques of these operations do not vary significantly for Hispanic patients, the ideals of physical beauty in Hispanic cultures are unique. These must be discussed before surgery and during surgical planning.

A Hispanic nose is typically characterized by thick nasal skin, a broad nasal base, and decreased projection from the rest of the face. Modification usually requires adding grafts to the tip or the top of the nose to strengthen the nose relative to the rest of the face.

Body contouring of the breast, abdomen, or trunk is guided by the patient's desires as always, but it is worth noting that buttock augmentation is more common in the Hispanic population because of societal preference for it. As discussed in the chapter on buttocks, this can be completed with an implant, a flap, or fat injection.

Skin with darker pigment is more likely to develop hypertrophic scarring or keloids and a loss of pigment. Hispanic patients and plastic surgeons must consider these risks before making a decision to undergo cosmetic surgery or skin resurfacing.

Aesthetic Surgery in Middle Eastern Patients

The cosmetic procedures selected by Middle Eastern patients are also in line with the cosmetic procedures desired by the general population, although typically more conservative. The most common procedures are liposuction and rhinoplasty (nose reshaping). The logistics are again the same, but to personalize to the patient's desires, these must be discussed before surgery and during surgical planning.

A Middle Eastern nose is also typically characterized by thicker skin, a broader base, and increased projection from the rest of the face. Modification usually requires more aggressive hump removal.

Body contouring of the breast, abdomen, or trunk is guided by the patient's desires, as always. Again, skin with darker pigment is more likely to develop poor scarring or pigmentation.